Ayurveda

How to Eat Well

Penny Spurr

Publication details
First Edition
ISBN
9781068551703 - paperback

Cover design by: Catherine Clarke

Disclaimer

This book is intended to provide information for educational purposes only. It is not intended to diagnose or treat any medical condition or illness. It is not a substitute for diagnosis or treatment prescribed by a healthcare professional. Always seek the counsel of your healthcare professional for health-related issues. The use of herbal supplements should be under the supervision of a trained practitioner.

Penny Spurr accepts no responsibility for the use or misuse of any information contained in this book. The author specifically disclaims any liability or loss, personal or otherwise, incurred as a consequence of the application of any of the content of this book.

The author assumes no responsibility or liability for any errors or omissions in the content of this book. Ayurveda is a personalised therapy that should be undertaken with a trained Ayurveda therapist (especially for anyone who is unwell or pregnant and for children and people aged over 65).

Contents

Part 1: Ayurveda

Foreword

by Cyrus Todiwala

When Penny Spurr approached me to write a foreword for her book, I was a bit surprised and thought what could I write for a book, I am not sure. But then she told me that it was on Ayurveda and it reminded me of a conversation we had a couple of years ago on the subject and at once my mind opened up.

Ayurveda is a subject quite dear to my heart, but not altogether followed by me as much as my father did. I grew up in a house where Dad was totally immersed in the subject and practised it wholeheartedly. I was highly asthmatic and suffered miserably as a child and many a medication was tried out on me. However, the simple basic Ayurvedic mixes did work and eventually an Ayurvedic doctor put me right. I can mention several of the many powders I was given and still do keep them to this day, just in case, but that is not all that this is about.

It's about understanding the body as Penny describes wholly. Ayurveda is not just whimsical, it is a study of the mind and body over five thousand years with the goal of a long and healthy life. My dad was a very fit ninety-seven-year-old and it was only a nasty fall that destroyed it all. He did not wish to be dependent on anyone so let himself go.

Dad referred to a book all the time, a book written in old fashioned Gujarati, and I have it with me now. I would love it translated, only it's too expensive and the book is very, very old. However, when I took my early plunge into pickle making, I used to call Dad about the spices I was blending, and, more often than not he would ask me to call him back. Then when I did, he would say that I cannot mix X with Y as that will give the person eating 'Vaa', i.e. bad wind meaning gas, or in other words indigestion. This taught me so much and we managed a good balance and still use that to this day with our chutneys and pickles.

So, what is Penny after? After doing her diploma in Ayurveda and being connected to the food industry, she decided to write a book on the benefits of Ayurveda on how to eat well following those principles.

It is not just interesting, but the topics are very much in keeping with how our bodies are exposed to a myriad of foods today, therefore leading to several ailments, which could be avoided. Ayurvedic herbal mixtures are widely available these days online and for many they are an alternative option to taking drugs, though understanding is necessary.

I am myself keen to re-explore more newfound knowledge and see how we can balance our lives better. Like my father, my son Jamsheed has immersed himself in this subject and I am thrilled to see all the small combinations that Dad made, and I do some for myself, which he never knew of but is practising. For me that is unbelievable and when you see a chip off the old block, you know that the junior Todiwala is on the right track with this mad world of ours where one is exposed to so many distractions in food that discipline goes out the window.

I wish her the very best and look forward to reading and comparing notes and hoping that it rekindles many memories for me besides helping the wider community and more specifically chefs today in understanding the human body and how we can serve our customers better.

Cyrus Rustom Todiwala OBE, DL,
celebrity television chef and Indian chef proprietor of Café Spice Namasté, London

Gratitude

I wish to thank the following people:

My teacher Vaidya Atreya Smith, Director of the European Institute of Vedic Studies. I am indebted to him for his generosity in sharing his vast wisdom, knowledge and experience of Ayurveda, especially in how to make the Classic Ayurveda teachings relevant and applicable in today's world and for writing the introduction to this book.

Sarah Williams (Medical Herbalist and Ayuverda Practitioner), Vic Laws MBE, Rod Cuff, and Katharine Smith of Heddon Publishing. I am so grateful for your kindness, time and generosity, I couldn't have done it without you.

I also wish to thank Cyrus Todiwala for generously writing the Foreword.

Introduction

by Vaidya Atreya Smith

Food is not only energy for the body, it also builds and maintains the tissues and structure of the body. Therefore, diet and the consumption of different food articles has a direct impact on our health. As Hippocrates said: “Let food be thy medicine and medicine be thy food.”

Ancient cultures from places such as Greece and India knew the value and effect of food on the body. Hence, they placed great emphasis on diet as part of their medical systems. Ayurveda, the traditional medical system of India, has never lost sight of the importance of diet in terms of health and longevity. Unlike the development of medicine in Europe and the West, nutrition has stayed as an integral part of the Indian medical system and is treated as a main treatment for health issues.

The Ayurvedic view is that diet (*ahara*) and exercise (*vihara*) are the pillars of health and form the basis of any treatment. Their comprehension is that no therapeutic treatment will work effectively if diet and exercise are not implemented as the foundation of the remedy. While Ayurveda has a wide range of diverse therapies ranging from external treatments with oil to complicated compounds of medicinal plants, diet and exercise remain the basis of any therapeutic approach.

These ancient medical systems are based on awareness that diet has a direct effect on health, and also that each person is unique and digests food differently. For example, the Greek and Indian systems developed methodologies to understand different types of digestive systems which are a reflection of metabolism as a whole. This understanding is the basis of Hippocrates famous dictum, “It is more important to know what sort of person has a disease than to know what sort of disease a person has.”

This understanding led to individual approaches to medical treatments vs ‘one size fits all’ treatments that are common in modern medicine. Our modern science has long been aware that there are vast differences between humans in terms of how they respond to environmental stimulus. The study of metabolic responses to drugs, environmental changes, and diseases is a new, promising area of metabonomic research. Metabolic fingerprints can be obtained by analytical techniques such as nuclear magnetic resonance (NMR). This research has shown that characterising individual metabolic fingerprints may allow researchers to (i) better plan personalised therapy and nutrition; (ii) better predict and assess drug efficacy and toxicity; (iii) follow phenotype changes as a function of disease progression; (iv) perform cost-effective screenings on large human populations, and (v) address how possible long-term changes may be related to aging (information downloaded from https://www.pnas.org by 81.13.228.108 on August 2, 2024).

While this is an important step forward in the development of personalised treatments in modern medicine, Ayurveda has always used this personalised approach in treatments. The wise sages (Rishis) developed a system of seven metabolic types in humans that could be subdivided into various subtypes. This methodology was developed over many generations by direct observation of humans in their environment and their interaction with different foodstuffs. These observations were codified into the present system.

Therefore, following dietary advice from the Ayurvedic system means understanding how the body will digest and use energy from food in different environmental conditions. The Indian system is not a means to classify people but rather a methodology in which to understand different metabolic responses to food and environmental changes. Unfortunately, this is not well understood in the West as Ayurvedic medicine was mainly introduced along with other Indian traditions such as yoga and meditation as a Wellness system.

The Indian system of medicine not only understood the importance of food as medicine and how this affected people differently, it also understood the effect of diet on the psychology. Some of the most ancient texts in India are the Upanishads, which come from the four Vedas. The Chāndogya Upaniṣaid, in verse 5.5.1, states the following understanding: "Food is divided into three parts in the body, the gross (sthūla) constituent becomes feces, the medium (madhyama) constituent becomes tissue, and the subtle (sūkṣma) constituent becomes mind."

This means that everything we eat will have non-nutritive components (e.g. fibre, etc.) that are evacuated, as well as nutritive components that form and maintain the body structure. In addition to this basic idea is the concept that food forms and influences the human psychology. Primarily this asserts the importance of eating fresh, whole food that is full not only of nutrients but also life itself.

This book, *Ayurveda - How to Eat Well* explains in simple terms how to use the Ayurvedic system in modern life and our current environment of excess. It is a valuable contribution to Ayurveda and modern nutrition in that it explains the system in simple terms that are easy to digest and understand.

Vaidya Atreya Smith, BSc, MS, is the Director of the European Institute of Vedic Studies and author of **Ayurveda Nutrition**

My Journey

This book is designed as an introduction both to Ayurveda and to how you can use the wisdom of Ayurveda to help you eat well.

The term 'Ayurveda' is derived from the Sanskrit words *Ayur* (life) and *Veda* (sacred science or knowledge). Thus, Ayurveda translates to 'knowledge of life'. It has a simple, elegant logic that is as relevant today as it was 3000 years ago. It covers a breadth of knowledge on how to live well and on healing the body.

This book is important for everyone who cooks and eats. It explains the principles of *Ahara Chikitsa* (Food as Medicine) and shows how to put this knowledge into practice for your own wellbeing.

This is not a recipe book, but it shows you how to incorporate the principles of Ayurveda into how you eat well. It's about how to create a personalised diet to make you feel more energised and alive. It emphasises using fresh, seasonal, local foods to cook meals that don't have to be expensive or complicated. It offers a fresh perspective on how to put nutrition into practice in a simple and logical way. In Part 1 we explore some of the classical principles of Ayurveda. In Part 2 we look at how this

applies to food, then in Part 3 we look at how to put this into practice.
I suggest you read the book in the order in which it's written, as fresh information builds on earlier information as we go along. It all interweaves and interconnects, so not until you've got to the end does it truly make sense as a whole.

A consultation with an Ayurveda practitioner usually focuses on advice tailored to our specific immediate needs; realistically, there is insufficient time to go into details about the principles of Ayurveda and how to eat well, but this book helps to fill that gap.

My background is in hospitality management and I'm a trained chef. Having trained at Westminster College in London, I spent the next ten years working as a hospital catering manager, including working at the Royal Marsden Cancer Hospital, St George's University Hospital, London, and the John Radcliffe Oxford University Hospital. It was there that I started to develop an interest in the relationship between diet and health. I moved to work in local authority catering, managing the catering in schools, colleges, care homes, day centres and meals on wheels. This gave me additional experience of feeding both younger and older people.

Much later, I moved to the New Forest in the south of England and retrained to work in healthcare, including working for the Alzheimer's Society and as a Macmillan Professional before retiring to nurse my own father, who had Parkinson's disease.

I now work as an Ayurveda Therapist and live with my Golden Retriever dog, and the best part of our day is walking in nature. I am also learning the ancient language of Sanskrit, the language of Ayurveda.

Nutrition is a relatively new science and over the last forty years much has changed. You followed the guidelines of the day only for these to be updated. This has left much confusion as to what is the correct dietary advice. It wasn't until I learnt about Ayurveda that I thought, 'Yes, this makes sense'. It has withstood the test of time, is based on an elegant logic and is not a 'one diet fits all' approach. Learning Ayurveda feels like the culmination of my life's work.

I was so fortunate to find Ayurveda in 2015 and was privileged to learn through the European Institute of Vedic Studies with Vaidya Atreya Smith. He taught the classic Ayurveda teachings and shared his experiences of how to apply these in the West, where we have a different climate, diet and heritage from that of India, where Ayurveda originated. I originally learnt for my own interest but when we got to the end of the two-year diploma course, which included time studying in India, he encouraged us to share this wisdom with others – and this book is my contribution. This is the book I originally looked for and couldn't find, so I thought, 'Well, perhaps I need to write it' – a short, easy-to-read, affordable introduction to Ayurveda, 'How to Eat Well' written from a practical cook's perspective.

So, what is so special about Ayurveda?

Firstly, it's not one size fits all; it recognises that we are all slightly different. We have different body frames; we have different characteristics, and we experience different types of illnesses. This is explained by the *Dosha – Vata, Pitta* and *Kapha.* As someone with a predominance of the Kapha Dosha, I have experienced having much more energy since I stopped eating breakfast and started selecting lighter meals. It's not just what you eat but how you eat. Ayurveda explains why this makes sense.

Ayurveda explains digestion; it is our *Agni,* our digestive fire, and we all digest food slightly differently. As a Kapha person I have a slow digestion, but through adding a few pungent and bitter spices to my daily diet and eating foods that suit my Dosha, my digestion now is the best it's ever been.

A few years ago, my partner Vic had a triple-bypass heart operation. The surgery sent his body into shock. He woke up in the Intensive Care Unit to a lunch of beef bourguignon, a heavy beef stew that is hard on the digestive system. Unsurprisingly his digestive system objected to this assault and shut down. There are times when a light, healing, convalescent diet (*Vikriti)* makes sense.

Ayurveda practitioners ask you to stick out your tongue so that they can look for the presence of *Ama*, toxic substances in the gut, and identify which Dosha is out of balance. Ayurveda understands that problems in the digestive system are the starting point of most disease in the body. When I first learnt this from my teacher, my tongue showed the presence of Ama along with recognisable symptoms of brain fog and fatigue. After following an anti-Ama diet and using a digestive herbal tea formula for several months, I felt better than I had in forty years.

For those who are interested, Ayurveda also has a spiritual thread to it, but nothing is more important than cooking with love. Even the simplest meals are better when cooked with love and care.

Ayurveda encourages us to examine what we are eating, the quality of the food, and how it makes us feel. Vic works as a hospitality consultant, and we regularly enjoy fine wining and dining events to celebrate the industry. I have to confess that often these experiences leave me feeling heavy and dull and, despite the great efforts the chef has put in to create some culinary masterpiece, unless I consciously limit what I eat and drink I can't digest it. One of the great exceptions to this is the chef Raymond Blanc at Le Manoir aux Quat' Saisons Hotel, just outside Oxford. The quality of the food is superb, the seasonal fruit and vegetables come from his own kitchen gardens, he and his team cook with passion and love that shine through into the finished dish, and he understands digestion. Last time we went there, the dinner included a divine risotto using fresh vegetables and herbs from the garden; it was a very small and light portion, tasted delicious and yet was so simple. I got up from the table that evening feeling energised, satisfied and happy. What joy!

Ayurveda doesn't have to be about eating Asian-style dishes. I was greatly inspired by a few days at the Ayurveda retreat the Clover Mill, founded by Julie Dent, in the Malvern Hills in Worcestershire. Most of the recipes were vegan, using *Sattvic* vegetables straight from the kitchen garden, making delicious Ayurveda meals with an English flavour to them. Ayurveda shows us the principles of how to create dishes that harmoniously blend textures (*Gunas*) and flavours (*Rasa*) to make them both culinary and gastronomic masterpieces. However, most of us don't just wake up one day and decide to change our diet unless there's a compelling reason to do so. It's a journey of continual little changes. Make one, see how you feel, and then try another. I am still doing this! I'm not perfect, I'm a 'work in progress'. Ayurveda inspires me to continue with my journey.

One of the most exciting things about Ayurveda is that it is as relevant today as it was in ancient times. Modern medicine, especially Functional Medicine, is now beginning to scientifically verify and prove that Ayurveda works, especially in the significance it gives to gut health. It just uses a modern scientific language instead of Sanskrit, the language of Ayurveda.

I hope you will enjoy reading this book and be inspired to put some of the recommendations into practice to support your own health.

Wishing you good health, vitality and joy.

Penny

Part 1: Ayurveda

1. Introduction to Ayurveda

What is Ayurveda?

Ayurveda is considered to be the oldest health care system in the world, some suggest going back 5000 years, and is the only one with a spiritual background. It is said to have originated from divine wisdom and the wisdom of nature that was given to and studied by the wise sages called Rishis, who lived in the Himalayas of Northern India. It has an oral tradition using the ancient Indian language of Sanskrit.

The word *Āyurveda* is made up of two Sanskrit words, *Āyur*, which in Sanskrit means life or longevity, and *Veda*, which means knowledge or sacred knowledge. It is often translated as the sacred science of health, medicine or longevity.

Ayurveda is still very much alive today in Southeast Asia and India, with clinics in both rural and urban settings. Most practitioners there who call themselves a 'doctor' are qualified as 'Western' Medical Doctors as well as in Ayurveda. Ayurveda is also kept alive in the homes of many families, where homely herbal remedies and the knowledge of how to eat well is passed down from one generation to the next. Today it is also starting to gain a larger international recognition. The most important and useful classic works of Ayurveda literature are the Caraka Smahita (500CE) and the Astanga Hrdayam (700CE), which are still in use today.

The goal is to achieve a long and healthy life. In Ayurveda perfect health is described as a balance between body, mind, spirit and social wellbeing. It is a traditional medicine that covers a breadth of knowledge on living well and healing the body. One of the main tenets is the emphasis on moderation, both in what we eat and in how we live our lives. This book introduces you to the Ayurveda Principles of Food as Medicine – Ahara Chikitsa.

Basic principles of Ayurveda

There are two core principles that are the cornerstones of Ayurveda.

1. The first is Karma, that 'All actions, words and deeds will result in a consequence and have an effect'. In Ayurveda we are aiming to keep the body in balance to achieve health; however, many of the actions and choices we make in terms of diet and lifestyle can have adverse consequences that throw the body out of balance. Every imbalance has a cause.

We seek to find and treat the cause of an imbalance rather than just treat the symptoms. For example, if you suffer from hyperacidity, you might take antacid medication to relieve the symptoms, but this by itself does not address the root cause of the problem.

2. The second principle is that 'Like increases like and opposites reduce'. If am cold and go to stand outside on a freezing cold day when it's wet and windy and eat ice-cream, I will get colder (like increases like). Conversely, 'opposites reduce and balance' – if I am cold and put on warm clothes, make a hot meal, have a mug of ginger tea, and go and sit by the fire, I will get warmer; this will reduce the feeling of cold and bring me back to balance.

Ayurveda Ahara Chikitsa – Food as Medicine

This book is all about using our diet and the food we eat as medicine or therapy to balance the body. In Sanskrit *Ahara* can be translated as food or diet, and *Chikitsa* means medicine, treatment or therapy, hence Ahara Chikitsa – Food as Medicine.

Ayurveda treats the individual by formulating a tailored dietary plan. We are all different and the ways in which we digest and metabolise food vary accordingly. Due to this, we all respond in contrasting ways to different food; it is not 'one diet fits all'. This book demonstrates the Ayurveda principles of how to identify your individual body type and how to eat to support your health.

Ahara Chikitsa demonstrates that food has both psychological and physiological effects and can be used to balance the physical, mental and emotional aspects of life. Think of the taste of a lemon; it's sour, light and sharp. In home-made lemonade it can be refreshing and awaken the mind (psychological); but in excess, lemons can create hyperacidity (physiological).

The therapeutic effect of food comes not just from the food itself but also from the way in which it is used: for instance, the time of day when food is eaten and whether it is raw or cooked. Is breakfast the most important meal or the least important? There isn't one right answer; it will depend on your individual body type.

Ahara Chikitsa also explains that how the body responds to food provides information on what caused the original problem; if you suffer from constipation, you will know that some foods help to solve the problem while others will exacerbate it.

Ayurveda encourages us to develop the capacity to observe – both ourselves and nature. Observing your body and how you respond to different foods with the understanding of Ayurveda gives you the tools to identify the cause of an imbalance and how to address it. Sometimes, simple changes to your diet can have a profound effect on how you feel.

Our connection with the natural world

Ayurveda was originally taught in nature: observing the world around us; the seasons; the plants. Shopping in supermarkets disconnects us from the world of nature; a simple example is noticing that some vegetables grow up towards the heat of the summer sun, such as runner beans, whilst others store and hide their goodness in the soil, such as carrots. We are not designed to be disconnected from nature; we feel good spending time in nature, especially when there is the opportunity to relax, let go and find peace.

Pancha Maha Bhutas – Five Great Elements

Pancha means five, *Maha* great, and *Bhuta* can be described as elements or categories of matter. These five great elements are: ether, air, fire, water and earth.

Elements	Sanskrit name
Ether or Space	Akasha
Air or Wind	Vayu
Fire	Agni
Water	Jala
Earth	Prthivi

Table 1.1 Pancha Maha Bhutas with their Sanskrit names

The origins of Ayurveda are linked to Indian Vedic philosophies. One of these is the Sankhya

Darshana, which describes the concept of creation. The Sankhya provides a beautifully logical way of describing how pure intelligent consciousness gave birth to creation, which includes the creation of all matter, the Pancha Maha Bhutas.

This concept identifies that cosmic energy manifests itself as the Pancha Maha Bhutas:

1. First is ether, the lightest element, which is the source of all matter and creates the empty space that provides the field of potential.
2. Second is air, the cause of wind and movement.
3. Third is fire, which is responsible for all transformation.
4. Fourth is water, which represents fluid matter and the principle of cohesion.
5. Fifth is earth, which relates to solidity and stability.

Within this concept each element contains some of the previous elements, for example earth contains mainly earth but also some of the previous four elements – ether, air, fire and water – to hold it together.

Absolutely everything can be classified using these categories of matter. These become the foundation building blocks for everything in life, ourselves, and the plant world. The Pancha Maha Bhutas are the foundation of Ayurveda.

Gunas – 20 Qualities

The *Gunas* (*Gurvadi Gunas*) are ten pairs of qualities that give us a way of understanding the universe; they describe everything in nature and give us a good idea of how different types of food will affect us. These pairs of Gunas act as opposites: e.g., hot versus cold, heavy versus light. They also work on a continuum – in this case, from very hot to warm to cool to very cold, and very heavy to very light. These Gunas come from the three Maha Gunas: Sattva, Rajas and Tamas.

Gunas	**Opposite Gunas**
Cold – Shita	Hot – Ushna
Wet/oily – Snigdha	Dry – Ruksha
Heavy – Guru	Light – Laghu
Gross – Sthula	Subtle – Sukshma
Dense – Sandra	Flowing – Drava
Static – Sthira	Mobile – Chala
Dull – Manda	Sharp – Tikshna
Soft – Mrudu	Hard – Kathina
Smooth – Shlakshna	Rough – Khara
Cloudy – Picchila	Clear – Vishada

Table 1.2 20 Gunas with their Sanskrit name

The Gunas are used to describe the Pancha Maha Bhutas (five great elements).

The first three pairs are the ones we work with most in Ayurveda:

- Ether is cold, light and dry.
- Air is dry and light.
- Fire is hot, dry and light.
- Water is wet/oily, heavy and cold.
- Earth is heavy, cold and dry.

Prana

Prana can be translated as our 'vital life force'. The term Prana is used in many different contexts – at its simplest it is pure energy, our source of life, and without it we die. We obtain Prana from our breath, sunlight, water and natural foods. Some foods such as grains and pulses require cooking to release this energy.

Three Maha Gunas – Sattva, Rajas and Tamas

Within the Vedic philosophy of Sankhya Darshana, the three *Maha Gunas – Sattva, Rajas and Tamas* – are an integral part of creation and everything is made from them, including the Pancha Maha Bhutas (ether, air, fire, water and earth). They are also used to describe our individual intellect (*Buddhi*). These concepts are used in Yoga and Hindu scriptures.

In Ayurveda our mental nature is observed according to Sattva, Rajas and Tamas. We have all three within us and every experience we have is made up of these same Maha Gunas. How we choose to live our lives will determine which of them is most dominant within us and influencing our state of mind.

Sattva

Sattva is the light of consciousness and relates to loving kindness, truth, right living and our spiritual purpose. According to Ayurveda the mind is pure Sattva before it becomes changed by the social conditioning of our Rajasic world. People who display Sattvic characteristics act with intelligence, express clarity of thought, are adaptable and harmonious, and take care of themselves. They see life as a learning experience and try to see the good in all people. They are peaceful people whose inner peace radiates out to those around them. We should aspire to having a Sattvic mind for our health and wellbeing, especially those of us on a spiritual path.

Rajas

Rajas is about action, creativity and our get-up-and-go. However, in excess it can create a defused energy and turbulence in the mind, which may be agitated by anxiety and disturbed thoughts. People who display Rajasic characteristics can become critical, dominating and self-centred, with a desire for more and new sensations, and are not content with what they have. Our fast-paced, consumer-oriented, social-media-driven twenty-first-century world is intrinsically Rajasic.

You will have seen people who can never sit still and are always busy doing things; these are Rajasic types. They attempt too much, expect too much, and overextend themselves. These people often have an inability to say ‘No’. Remember that by saying no when it is appropriate you are also protecting your immune system. Sometimes this inability to say no can be a fear of missing out, whereas it can sometimes be empowering to say no, and other people should respect you for that.

It can often be difficult to give ourselves permission to just sit still and do nothing. It’s as if it’s a crime or we feel guilty if we’re not pushing ourselves forward and looking outwards all the time. We have forgotten that this is not necessarily good for us. A lot of people find meditation very difficult because their mind is jumping around too much.

Tamas

Tamas is the energy of darkness, rest and calm; without Tamas we would not sleep. However, in excess it can reflect a mind drowned by negativity, depression, self-destructive behaviour, dishonesty and inertia. When we are under the influence of Tamas, we see others as being the enemy and our capacity to challenge wrong and right, bad and good, is taken over by lethargy.

When we finally become exhausted from our Rajasic world we can spill over into Tamas. Tamas attracts misery and suffering. We can see this in our current mental health crisis (including depression and addiction) as well as in criminality and violence.

This is a very difficult place in which to find yourself and, because it makes you feel so heavy and lethargic, it is difficult to get yourself out of it. In order to do so, people in this place need others to help them, to show them where they are and to give them easy steps, taken one at a time, that are not too difficult for them.

When ill, they often do not seek proper treatment and have a devitalised diet. They will often accept their disease as fate and will not help themselves.

Those in a Tamasic state must progress through Rajas before they can reach Sattva, so it is the action of Rajas that will help them to move forward.

These Maha Gunas are not fixed, and the good news is that we can work on ourselves to cultivate the more positive characteristics of each of them. We may develop Sattva through yoga practice, meditation, contemplation and prayer. We can also foster Sattva through being compassionate, showing integrity, and being of service to others.

Additional factors that can help us with increasing Sattva include spending more time in nature, pursuing creative activities, and building a life in harmony with one's Dosha constitution. These habits all help to build more Sattva in our lives. However, we need to be careful because in our Rajasic world even something like yoga can become highly competitive and forced, which is not how it was designed.

In Ayurveda the effect of eating different types of food will influence our mental balance and behaviour as well our physical health and wellbeing. Foods express the attributes of Sattva, Rajas and Tamas.

2. Doshas

Doshas – Vata, Pitta and Kapha

The Doshas are a concept unique to Ayurveda. They are said to come from Prana. This is a brief overview of what they are in relation to Ahara Chikitsa (Food as Medicine). For those of us more familiar with the Western understanding of anatomy and physiology, the concept of the Doshas can be difficult to get our heads around. For simplicity, we can view the Doshas as a metaphor to describe the human body, its characteristics and functions. The Sanskrit word *Dosha* translates as 'a fault', so Doshas are also seen as the cause of imbalance and disease in the body.

According to Ayurveda, the body is made up of three Doshas – *Vata, Pitta* and *Kapha.*

There are four key points that are important to understanding the Doshas:

1. Doshas are made up of the Pancha Maha Bhutas.

Our bodies are made from all the Pancha Maha Bhutas (elements), but each of us has a unique combination of these elements.

• Vata people have a predominance of ether and air.
• Pitta people have a predominance of fire and water.
• Kapha people have a predominance of water and earth.

These elements show up in the body as both physical and psychological traits. We most notably see this in the structure of the body; Vata people usually have thin bodies, Pitta people have a medium build and Kapha people often have bigger and stronger bodies.

2. Doshas control and manage how the body works. Doshas manage all the functions of the body to maintain balance and health.
• Vata manages everything to do with movement.
• Pitta manages all transformation, including digestion.
• Kapha manages cohesion, lubrication and stability.

3. Doshas identify the health of the body.
When we are balanced, healthy and feeling well, this state is called *Prakriti*; when we are out of balance or unwell, it is called *Vikriti.* The body works intelligently to regulate and keep this Prakriti balance. However, the very act of living with our diet, lifestyle and climate can throw us out of balance; even a bad night's sleep can unbalance us and cause Vikriti.

4. The Gunas are used to describe the Doshas. Each of the Pancha Maha Bhutas (elements) has identifiable Gunas (qualities). For example, wind and movement create lightness and dryness (visualise drying washing outside on the clothes-line and so changing the clothes from being heavy and wet to being light and dry). Therefore, as we can see in Table 2.1 below, each Dosha has distinctive Gunas that correspond with its elements.

Vata	**Elements:** Ether (space) and air (wind) **Function:** Movement **Gunas (qualities):** Dry, light, cold, rough and mobile
Pitta	**Elements:** Fire and water **Function:** Transformation and digestion **Gunas (qualities):** Slightly oily, penetrating, hot, light and spreading
Kapha	**Elements:** Earth and water **Function:** Cohesion, stability and lubrication **Gunas (qualities):** Oily, cool, heavy, slow and static

Table 2.1 Elements, Function and Gunas (qualities) that relate to each Dosha

Doshas and nature's rhythm

The Doshas have a natural rhythm and work in harmony with time: the seasons of the year, the time of the day and as we age.

When we are in balance and healthy (Prakriti), the Doshas function with intelligence, creating health and harmony. Like waves in the sea, the Doshas follow a natural rhythm; as one Dosha increases, another reaches its peak and the third is reducing and hopefully goes back to where it started.

When we are out of balance (Vikriti), the Doshas get disturbed and lose their intelligence and rhythm, causing disruption; the peak becomes aggravated and goes too high or the Dosha doesn't fully reduce back to where it started, and this eventually causes disease. The Doshas find natural balance by attracting their opposite Gunas (qualities). When out of balance, a Dosha will sabotage itself with things that increase it. We see a clear example of this in addictions, for instance to alcohol or chocolate.

Balancing and correcting Dosha function is the basic aim and goal of treatment within Ayurveda. The main thrust is to determine the Dosha that is causing the Vikriti imbalance or disease and treat this with Ahara Chikitsa (Food as Medicine), lifestyle therapies and medicinal herbs in order to take the Dosha back to its original Prakriti balance and health. This model is based on the idea that by increasing the intelligence of the body it will function correctly.

Doshas and function

Doshas can be used to describe how our bodies function.

Vata Dosha is responsible for the function of all movement in the body. Vata is the master Dosha and is responsible for breathing, speech, muscular movement, elimination of bodily waste, the movement of digestion and the nervous system.

Pitta Dosha is responsible for the function of fire and transformation in the body. It governs heat and light in the body, including transformation of the food we eat through digestion, and the function of the heart, liver and eyesight. It is also the energy that creates heat in the body: our temperature.

Kapha Dosha is responsible for everything to do with cohesion and stability in the body. It lubricates the joints, brain, lungs, heart, mucous membranes and digestion. It gives a sense of taste and provides the body with stability, strength and balance.

Dosha Prakriti

Dosha Prakriti is your individual Dosha profile of how much Vata, Pitta and Kapha you have in your body. You are made up of all three Doshas; however, most of us show a predominance of one or two Doshas that define the physical and mental characteristics we were born with. It is your unique genetic blueprint. It identifies who you are from birth and does not change – it is your 'normal'. It identifies your state of balance and health and enables you to recognise your unique style of functioning in the world. You have your parents to thank for who you are, as it reflects their health and lifestyle factors at the time of your conception.

Now, it may be that there are aspects of yourself that you would like to change; for example, many people are not happy with their body weight. Vata people often have difficulty putting on weight and Kapha people often have difficulty reducing their weight. However, you must be realistic and work within the parameters of your Dosha Prakriti and find a healthy balance for your body type.

It is of great value to honour and recognise what your Dosha Prakriti is – because you can't change it. It is as it is, and it is always what you have to go back to. When you can accept that this is who you are, you can learn to work with it to balance your health and wellbeing, bringing a sense of acceptance and peace for yourself and others.

Dosha Prakriti characteristics

The characteristics of the three Doshas come from the elements of which they are made. We have all three Doshas within us, which is necessary for the functioning of the body; however, the mix of the

Pancha Maha Bhutas (elements) often shows a predominance of one or two Doshas.

These characteristics have been observed and identified over hundreds of years and give us a stereotypical pen-picture for each Dosha.

- Vata Prakriti types often have a thin, light body, and are quick, lively and changeable with a variable appetite and digestion. Vata are the air people; they often have an artistic temperament, are full of ideas and creativity and go beyond the limits of conformity.

- Pitta Prakriti types normally have a medium-sized body with average strength and endurance. They have a strong digestion, a sharp intellect, competitive nature and strong willpower. Pitta are the fire people; they are the managers and are good at solving problems.

- Kapha Prakriti types often have a larger body with good strength and endurance. They tend to be steady and reliable with slow speech and digestion. They are calming, grounded and compassionate. Kapha are the earth and water people, motivated by family and security.

Use the Dosha questionnaire in Appendix 1 to determine your Dosha Prakriti. When using the Dosha questionnaire, try to avoid being overly persuaded by these pen-pictures or personal bias. It is not always easy to identify your own Dosha balance, especially when this is mixed with Vikriti. The Vata–Kapha Dosha mix especially can sometimes be mistaken for a Pitta Dosha; Vata and Kapha in many ways are opposites and people with this mix can be highly successful, but just have a different take on life to that of a Pitta person.

Dosha Vikriti

Dosha Vikriti identifies the Doshas when they are imbalanced. Vikriti translates as 'changed, altered or diseased'; it is when your Prakriti is covered up or obscured by imbalances. It is when you are out of balance, ill or in pain, which covers up and distorts how you normally are in health, both physically and mentally.

Vikriti arises from an incorrect relationship with our environment through diet, lifestyle and climate. Our modern lives are full of stress and stimulation that can produce Vikriti. It is a state of the mind and body in which the individual is more prone to disease because the Doshas are aggravated and increased.

Any or all of the Doshas can become imbalanced. It is usually your strongest Dosha that goes out of balance first, although our modern way of living creates a predominance of Vata aggravation. The goal of Ayurveda is to treat the Dosha imbalance and take it back to the Prakriti balance with which you were born. Diet and lifestyle changes are very important in order to return to your personal Dosha balance or Prakriti.

Dosha Vikriti characteristics

When the Doshas are imbalanced, the Gunas (qualities) become increased and aggravated, showing exaggerated characteristics to those of Prakriti. Again, these can give us a stereotypical pen-picture for each Dosha.

- Vata Vikriti – When aggravated, Vata can become erratic, anxious, fearful, exhausted and ungrounded. This can lead to complications such as constipation, dry skin, joint pain, insomnia, throbbing pain and arthritis, as well as problems with our mental health. Improper eating habits, over-exercise and excessive worry, dry cold weather, early mornings and late afternoons, strong winds and travel can all increase Vata.

- Pitta Vikriti – When aggravated, Pitta can become hot-headed and sharp, irritable, angry and achievement-oriented workaholics. This can lead to inflammatory disorders, skin problems, heart problems, acid reflux, diarrhoea and repressed emotions. Improper eating habits, insufficient sleep, indulgence in hot emotions, midday and midnight and summer sun can all increase Pitta.

- Kapha Vikriti – When aggravated, Kapha can become depressed, lethargic, resistant to change, sleepy and inactive. This can lead to overeating and weight gain, congestion in the lungs and sinuses, slow digestion and fluid retention. Improper eating habits, sleeping during the day, rainy and cloudy weather, late winter and early spring can all increase Kapha.

Use the Dosha questionnaire in Appendix 1 to determine your Dosha Vikriti as it is now today.

Doshas and their Gunas (qualities)

Each Dosha can be characterised by its Gunas. Using the principle of 'like increases like and opposites reduce', we use Gunas of the opposite qualities to balance and reduce the Doshas. Once you understand your individual Dosha make-up you can use this information to keep your body in balance.

- Vata Dosha – has the qualities of cold, dry, light, subtle, mobile, sharp, hard, rough and clear. This shows up in both physical and mental characteristics: for example, cold hands and feet, coarse dry hair, a light body frame and dry, rough skin. The opposite Gunas are used to treat aggravated Vata – warm, oily and unctuous food.

- Pitta Dosha – has the qualities of hot, humidly oily/slightly wet, light, subtle, flowing, spreading, sharp, soft and smooth. This shows up in warm hands and feet, a sharp mind and smooth, oily skin.

Using the same principle, Pitta aggravation is reduced by cooler and drier food.

• Kapha Dosha – has the qualities of cool, humidly oily/wet, heavy, gross, static, dull, soft, smooth and cloudy. This shows up as a larger and heavier body frame, abundant oily hair, cool skin and a slow and steady methodical temperament. Hot, dry and light foods are most useful to reduce Kapha, as these foods counteract Kapha's cool, wet and heavy Gunas.

How Doshas relate to time

The Doshas are not static; they are always changing and fluctuating. When the Doshas act with intelligence, they self-regulate and work in harmony for a dynamic balance. The goal of Ayurveda is to keep the body and mind in this dynamic balance; so, we use these natural cycles to create healthy lifestyle and dietary routines to keep the Doshas balanced and healthy to compensate for the imbalances in today's world.

Doshas in relation to seasons of the British year

As with all living things, the seasons of nature have a Prakriti, so the Doshas harmonise with the seasons. This table shows when the Doshas are at their highest peak and most aggravated.

Dosha	Peak season
Vata	Autumn (Fall)
Kapha	Spring
Pitta	Summer

Table 2.2 Dosha peaks in relation to the seasons of the British year

Vata starts to increase in late summer, reaches its peak in autumn and early winter and then starts to decrease again as we head towards late winter and early spring, when the weather starts to warm up again. When weather is cooler and windier, this can provoke Vata Dosha.

Kapha starts to increase in late winter, reaches its peak in early spring when the earth starts to warm up, then decreases again in late spring, when it starts to melt away into Pitta season. It is a time of growth, when we often get a lot of wet and colder weather that can aggravate Kapha Dosha.

Pitta starts to increase in late spring, reaches its peak in summer, and then starts to decrease again as we head towards autumn. The heat of summer is most provoking for Pitta Dosha.

However, with climate change the weather is becoming more variable. It is not always possible to be precise as to when one season ends and another begins. We also see short periods of unseasonal changes and need to adjust our diet accordingly.

Ayurveda encourages us to eat what is grown locally and in season as this will balance the Doshas. As a general guideline we want to be eating:

- Vata diet in autumn and early winter
- Kapha diet in late winter and early spring
- Pitta diet in late spring and summer.

Using the principle of 'like increases like and opposites reduce', these Dosha diets focus on the foods that have the opposite Gunas (qualities) to the Dosha and therefore will reduce and balance the Dosha.

Seasonal diet for mixed Dosha types

This is an equally valid approach if your Dosha Prakriti is more or less equal in two of the Doshas:
- Vata/Pitta types – follow a Vata diet in autumn and winter and a Pitta diet in the spring and summer.
- Vata/Kapha types – follow a Vata diet in the summer and autumn and a Kapha diet in the winter and spring.
- Pitta/Kapha types – follow a Pitta diet in summer and autumn and a Kapha diet in winter and spring.

Doshas in relation to the time of day

The Doshas also have a daily cycle. Table 2.3 shows the cycles of time throughout the day when each Dosha peaks and becomes aggravated.

Vata	**Kapha**	**Pitta**
2am – 6am	6am – 10am	10am – 2pm
2pm – 6pm	6pm – 10pm	10pm – 2am

Table 2.3 Doshas in relation to the time of day

As we can see, Vata Dosha reaches a natural peak twice a day, between the hours of 2 and 6 (am and pm), and likewise for the other two Doshas, with Pitta reaching a peak between 10 and 2 (am and pm) and Kapha between 6 and 10 (am and pm). This gives us a guide as to how to live well, including when best to eat for each Dosha.

Sunrise to mid-morning is the time when Kapha is at its highest in all of us, when the weather is often cool and moist. In Ayurveda we are encouraged to rise and start our day before Kapha time, because otherwise we may be tempted to just lounge in bed.

By mid-morning the sun is rising and the day is getting warmer, bringing us into Pitta time. This is often when we have the greatest energy and are most productive. By mid-day the sun is at its highest point and has burnt off that early morning mist; this is when our digestion is strongest.

As we head towards mid-afternoon, we've used up that Pitta energy and it is now time to reduce our sensory stimulation and physical exercise, come in and enjoy a cup of herbal tea and perhaps do something creative. This is when Vata is most unstable.

Then at sunset we move into the Kapha night cycle. It's a time to slow down, calm the mind and prepare the body for sleep, as the sun gives way to darkness. We should ideally be in bed before 10 pm and the start of the Pitta night cycle. Our bodies are designed to rest at this time, and we should avoid the temptation to do anything other than sleep during these hours; otherwise Pitta gets a second wind, causing insomnia. Good-quality sleep is essential for our health. The Vata night cycle is early morning to sunrise, the Golden Hour, a time to rise and gently prepare ourselves for another day. These small hours of the early morning can be unsettling for Vata if our sleep is disturbed by restlessness.

Doshas and the cycle of life

The Doshas also relate to our age and the cycle of life. Childhood relates to Kapha, when children are growing and building their bodies. Pitta relates to our adult years when we have a fire in our belly for our careers and passions in life. Vata relates to our senior years, when we hopefully have more time for introspection and for enjoyment of a calmer pace of life. Although this doesn't change our Dosha Prakriti, it's helpful to consider this when planning our diet.

Dosha	Age
Kapha	0–15
Pitta	15–55
Vata	55+

Table 2.4 Doshas and the cycle of life

Childhood – Kapha time of life: 0–15 years

Childhood is the Kapha stage of life, when children are growing and developing fast and often experience mucus problems such as colds and ear problems, which are typical Kapha imbalances. Paediatrics is a specialism within Ayurveda.

Adulthood – Pitta time of life: 15–55 years (approximately)

Then we move into the Pitta time of life, when there is more fire in the belly. We move away from dependence on family and school and become more independent, building our careers and businesses. Many of us become more driven during this stage. Understanding the principles of a Pitta diet is helpful in navigating this period of our lives.

Senior years – Vata time of life: from about age 55 years and onwards

Moving into the senior years, we need to consider following a more Vata diet and the whole concept of Vata management. As we become more Vata, everything becomes drier; we become more tissue-deficient and more anxious. By following a Vata diet we can change this and help to make our later years healthier. It is important at this time of life to be mindful to eat less food, and to eat foods that are more easily digested. It is also during this time we hopefully have more time to spend on meditation, on introspection and finding wisdom in life.

Vata management – Dinacharya – are Ayurveda lifestyle therapies to help calm the mind and nourish the body. They include Abhyanga (oil massage), Pranayama (breathing exercises) and meditation. As we get older, hopefully we have more time to devote to these routines that ground and balance us.

Sātmya – Heritage

Satmya is the principle of habituation and our ability to adapt to our environment. We are predisposed to our place of origin, local foods, climate, habits and culture. We can struggle to adapt to changes brought about by moving to new foreign environments, or adapting to imported or modern foods that are not part of our heritage.

Where we were born in the world and the foods from our heritage will influence our diet. Living a life disconnected from the foods that our ancestors ate, moving to a new country and climate, introducing new foods or trying to drop a habit too quickly may create imbalance and stress.

We live in a world where many people travel and move from one country to another for work or a vacation or to emigrate. For many of us it is easy to get on an aeroplane and within hours be in a completely different country. It can be exciting to taste the foods of different cultures, but that is not to say that they will always agree with us. This doesn't just apply to where we were born; look at how the food we eat has changed in the last hundred years – it often bears little relation to the food eaten by our ancestors. It takes time for our digestive system to adjust to new foods and ways of eating.

According to the classical texts, we are designed to eat according to our heritage. Rice is the main grain grown and eaten in India and it is used traditionally in Ayurveda cookery, but it may not necessarily be appropriate for people from other parts of the world who have not always eaten large amounts of rice.

To eat an Ayurveda diet does not mean that you have to adopt an Indian vegetarian diet. This goes against the principles of Ayurveda and might cause long-term difficulties. Again, this emphasises the importance of eating seasonal foods that are locally grown. This does not just apply to food but also to other habits and adaptations: for example, the way you may have to adapt your sleep pattern if you do shift work around the clock can be challenging. With time, we can adapt and acquire new habits, including healthier ways of eating.

3. Agni, Ama and Mala

Agni – digestive fire

In Ayurveda the Sanskrit word *Agni*, which means fire, is used to describe digestion: the transformation, absorption and assimilation of both food and experiences. Experiences relate to how we respond to what is going on in our lives, what we see and hear, our thoughts and emotions.

Agni is managed by the Doshas; balancing and correcting Dosha function is how we manage digestion in the body.

We often take our digestion for granted, not questioning whether it is in balance or not. However, it is the foundation of good health. Just as we need to maintain a car and keep it filled with the correct fuel for it to run efficiently, the same is true with our bodies.

Functions of Agni

Agni converts food into energy for the body to function. We need an efficient Agni to have a fully functioning immune system.

It is responsible for processing information into knowledge or wisdom. Agni in the brain must burn brightly to enable us to digest our experiences in life and convert them into a healthy mental state.

It manages warmth in the body, giving a good colour to the skin and good circulation. We can see healthy Agni function through shiny hair, bright eyes and clear skin. Agni also gives strength to the tissues, bones and muscles.

It imparts cheerfulness and happiness and gives 'a spark to your life', providing the courage to face life and the experiences that come our way. When Agni is low it is difficult to find the energy and enthusiasm to cope with all the challenges in life.

The digestive process

The typical duration of digestion – that is, food passing through the gastrointestinal tract – depends on the state of our Agni, our Dosha balance and what we eat. Heavy foods such as red meat take much longer to digest than do light foods such as fruit. This process of digestion is broken down into three stages and correlates with the modern concept of digestion.

1. Stage one takes place in the mouth and upper stomach and is controlled by Kapha, which lubricates the mouth and gastrointestinal tract. This allows us to taste and swallow our food and protects the gastric mucous membrane.

2. Stage two takes place in the lower stomach and the small intestines and is controlled by Pitta. It is a fiery, acid environment and produces digestive enzymes to digest and break down the food, protein, fats and carbohydrates into usable chemicals that can be absorbed into the body to create energy.

3. Stage three takes place in the colon and is controlled by Vata. This is where absorption and assimilation of water and micronutrients (vitamins and minerals) and elimination take place.

Although all three Doshas are present throughout the body, they each have a primary site or ‘home’: for Vata it is the colon, Pitta the small intestines and Kapha the stomach. It is in these sites where the Doshas will first show signs of any imbalance or Vikriti.

Digestion by taste

Ayurveda identifies six tastes in food: sweet, sour, salt, pungent, bitter and astringent. These tastes correlate with the three Doshas. This concept has profound implications for our health that go way beyond whether we like a taste or not.

In Ayurveda the movement of food through the digestive system is described in terms of phases that are governed by each of the six tastes. This concept is unique to Ayurveda and is considered to reflect the order in which we digest food, starting with the sweet taste and finishing with the astringent taste.

- Kapha controls the sweet taste.
- Pitta controls the sour, salt and pungent tastes.
- Vata controls the bitter and astringent tastes.

Subtle digestion

Subtle digestion is the process of nourishing each tissue layer (*Dhatu*) of the body in a well-defined order. This model of subtle digestion demonstrates that we are made up of what we eat and absorb, because this actually makes our body tissues.

Once food has completed the digestive process in the gastrointestinal tract and waste has been eliminated from the body, what is left is nutrient fluid (*Ahara Rasa*). This fluid is then carried to each of the body tissue layers, which are fed and nourished in the following order:

1. Lymph/plasma (*Rasa* Dhatu)
2. Blood/haemoglobin (*Rakta* Dhatu)
3. Muscle (Mamsa Dhatu)
4. Fat (Meda Dhatu)
5. Bone (*Asthi* Dhatu)
6. Bone marrow and nerve tissue (*Majja* Dhatu)
7. Reproductive tissue (*Shukra* Dhatu)

One way to describe how subtle digestion nourishes these tissue layers is through an analogy with irrigation: an irrigation channel full of water nourishes each row of crops, with the nearest crops receiving water first and the crops at the end receiving water the last. In this same way, the nutrient fluid is carried from one body tissue to the next in its proper order. So, the first tissue to be fed by any food is plasma and the last is the reproductive tissue.

According to Ayurveda the entire process of digestion – of feeding these layers of body tissue – takes about 36 days, approximately 5 days for each tissue layer to be fed when the Agni is good and efficient. The end result of feeding all the tissues is the creation of *Ojas* – the most refined by-product of digestion, which can be defined as the subtle energy of our immune system.

Types of Agni

Digestion is multi-layered and doesn't just happen in the gastrointestinal tract; a more refined level of digestion happens at each stage within the functioning of the body. There are thirteen sources of Agni:

- One from the stomach – the main site of digestion is the stomach and small intestine (*Jathara Agni*)
- Five from the liver – digestion in the liver (*Pancha Bhuta Agni*) is associated with each of the five elements

• Seven from body tissues – each of the seven body tissues (*Dhatu*) has its own Agni.

Dosha digestion and Agni

Balanced Agni – a balanced Agni is what we are aiming for, with perfectly balanced Doshas and Agni leading to a healthy appetite and no digestive complaints. This is evidenced by faeces that float just under the water line in the toilet bowl. However, in reality the Doshas can easily become imbalanced, and this will change the state of our digestive fire. Overeating, emotional issues, poor food choices, seasonal changes and eating at the wrong time of the day are all factors that can interfere with our digestion.

• Vata Dosha – People with a predominant Vata Dosha tend to have a variable appetite. This can result in either snacking and grazing or forgetting to eat, unless they consciously eat three regular meals a day. When Vata Dosha becomes imbalanced, their digestive fire can become more variable (*Vishama Agni*), fluctuating between high and quick to low and slow, just like the wind can go from being very blustery to very still. This can result in bloating, wind, constipation, a sensitive digestive system, food intolerances and in some cases alternate diarrhoea and constipation.

• Pitta Dosha – People with a predominant Pitta Dosha tend to have a strong digestion, can digest most foods, become hungry quickly, and rarely miss a meal. However, when the digestive fire goes too high (*Tikshna Agni*) this can lead to hyperacidity, diarrhoea, high blood sugar and inflammation.

• Kapha Dosha – People with a predominant Kapha Dosha tend to have a slow steady digestion, need the least amount to eat, but love their food! When the Agni is aggravated, this can make the digestive fire lower and slower (*Manda Agni*), which can result in a sluggish digestion, diabetes, weight gain, excess mucus, fluid retention, tiredness and lethargy.

Microbiome

The human microbiome is made up of trillions of microorganisms, including bacteria, fungi and viruses that naturally inhabit the body, especially in the gut, our gastrointestinal system. They are essential for our health and support our digestion, immunity, brain and many other aspects of our health. A healthy microbiome has a very wide range of bacteria that comes from eating a varied diet of fresh seasonal wholefoods, vegetables, fruit, whole grains and beans. A diet lacking variety and high in processed foods or sugar; not having enough sleep; taking antibiotics or feeling stressed can combine to create an unhealthy microbiome with only a narrow range of bacteria. This weakens our gut and our immunity, making us more prone to allergies, illness and disease. We are only as healthy as our microbiome. In Ayurveda it is considered that most disease starts in the gastrointestinal tract.

Ama (toxins)

Ama is the Ayurveda term used to describe failed digestion: undigested food that accumulates in the digestive tract because of the failure of Agni, our digestive fire. It is caused by an inability to transform and assimilate food and eliminate waste products.

Ama is formed in the gastrointestinal tract where the undigested food stagnates and putrefies. If left untreated it will then enter the bloodstream and travel into deeper body tissues. If there is some level of indigestion, there will be some degree of Ama. This undigested food creates toxins in the body that upset the gut's intestinal flora, weaken the immune system, and eventually cause disease.

According to Ayurveda, all illness begins with Ama, excluding genetic diseases, accidents and trauma.

Causes of Ama

Ama will be formed in the body if both the Doshas and Agni (digestive fire) are imbalanced. This is in line with the thought in Western medicine that about 70% of our immune system is in the gut. The state of our Agni is the key to the health of our immune system.

Ama is created by eating too much food, eating at the wrong time, inappropriate food choices and stress. Inappropriate choices include eating too much red meat, other heavy foods, and overly refined or processed foods, especially those that contain agrochemicals. Some of us will also have individual trigger foods, such as wheat and dairy produce.

Ama is caused by the disruption of Agni, but this does not happen overnight; it is a slow accumulation, drop by drop over time, one meal at a time. According to Ayurveda it is this accumulation of Ama in the body, often over a long period of time, that is the starting point of disease.

Signs of Ama

Signs that Ama is present:

- digestive problems – indigestion, wind, bloating, diverticulitis and irritable bowel syndrome
- a coated tongue – especially first thing in the morning before brushing your teeth or using a tongue scraper
- exhaustion – lack of energy, brain fog, depression
- headache, migraine, aches and pains
- colds, fever
- allergies – up to three million people in the UK have a food allergy

• lack of taste and appetite
• stickiness of faeces, which tend to sink because they are heavy
• foul odours – breath, sweat, urine, faeces.

It is important to remove Ama, as left untreated it can go on to develop into serious health issues and disease.

Mala – faeces, urine and sweat

The three primary waste materials of the body are:

1. faeces (*Purisha*)
2. urine (*Mutra*)
3. sweat (*Sveda*).

The *Malas* are a normal by-product of the body. As with our digestive system, we often take the state of our bodily waste for granted, but this is an important factor in maintaining good health by clearing and cleaning the body. It is recommended to observe your faeces and urine every day to establish whether they are healthy or not. When the Malas are imbalanced, they act like Ama (toxins) and can cause disease.

Faeces

Defecation is necessary to expel undigested food and waste products from the body as faeces. For health we should defecate at least once a day, ideally in the morning. The colour, smell and texture of the faeces will depend on what we have eaten and the state of our Agni.

Faeces should ideally have the shape and consistency of a ripe banana that floats just under the surface of the toilet water. Too much undigested earth element and Ama can cause them to sink, too much undigested ether and air can cause them to float, and smelly faeces can be from undigested fire or an indication of Ama.

Imbalance can be caused by a range of factors, including food that is too heavy or light, too little exercise, eating too little fibre in our diet, excess use of laxatives or colonics, excessive travel, coffee, medication and stress.

• Vata Dosha – the faeces have a tendency to dryness with lower quantity. When imbalanced the faeces can be dry and hard like rabbit droppings or irregular, varying from very hard to very soft.

• Pitta Dosha – the faeces have a tendency to be strong smelling, looser and oily with medium quantity. When imbalanced the faeces can be very soft, even liquid, and can be quite smelly.

• Kapha Dosha – the faeces have a tendency to be oily with large, well-formed stools. When imbalanced the faeces are soft, sticky and pale in colour.

When an imbalance is not treated it can go on to cause more serious health issues, including blockages from diverticulitis or cancer. Constipation is a common problem in today's world and creates Ama. Constipation should be taken seriously, especially in the elderly, as it can have serious health implications. Faeces can also highlight other health issues in the body; black faeces can be an indication of the presence of blood; greenish-yellow can be an indication of problems in the liver, bile or gallstones.

In Ayurveda examination of the stool is by physical characteristics such as colour, quantity, odour and consistency. The National Health Service (NHS) Bristol Stool Chart is a modern way of using the faeces as a diagnostic aid, where we are aiming for a Type 4 stool that is soft and floating. (*See 'other links' in the bibliography*.)

Urine

The kidneys make urine by filtering wastes and excess water from the blood. It then passes to the bladder, which can hold about half a litre for two to five hours prior to urination. Urine should ideally be the colour of pale straw, clear, odourless and plentiful.

A range of factors, including drinking too little or too much fluid, a poor non-diverse gut microbiome, diuretic drugs, alcohol and fear can all adversely affect the health of our urine.

It is healthy to evacuate urine frequently during the day; a build-up of urine can result in bladder pain and water retention which, if left unchecked, can cause health issues including urinary tract infections, dehydration and incontinence. Urine can also highlight other health issues in the body, including diabetes and kidney disease.

Sweat

Some of us, especially Pitta types, sweat more than others. Sweat helps to regulate the body temperature, especially when we are hot, as well as removing waste through the skin, which is the largest organ of the body. A lack of salt, too much or too little exercise and the excessive use of heat therapies such as saunas can damage the normal function of sweat. Health concerns linked to sweat include itchy skin, high body temperature and fever.

Part 2: Food

4. Rasa: Taste

The Sanskrit word for taste is *Rasa*. Ayurveda identifies six tastes in foods: sweet, sour, salt, pungent, bitter and astringent. Ayurveda recommends that, ideally, we should eat all six tastes at every meal.

Rasa or taste is experienced firstly from the taste buds on the tongue as we eat. Smell and taste are closely linked, as the nerves in the nose identify smell. Both taste and smell are communicated to the brain, which processes the information on taste and smell as flavour. This function of taste is controlled by Vata. If Vata is imbalanced this communication malfunctions, resulting in digestion disturbances.

Through taste we can understand the substance of the food we are eating and therefore what it will do. Rasa shows us the Pancha Maha Bhutas (elements) and Gunas (qualities) in the tastes of food and is an indication of its properties and the chemical response expected from digestion.

The strength of taste is on a spectrum from very mild to very strong, depending on the individual food substance, climate and growing conditions. For example, the sweet taste goes from the extreme sweetness of white sugar with no nutrients through to the more neutral bland tastes of proteins, fats and carbohydrates in meat, milk and bread at the other end of the spectrum.

Our experience of taste affects our physical bodies, but it also has an effect on our mind and emotions. 'Sweet' is a happy taste and is one of the reasons why we often reach for something sweet if we are feeling bored, lethargic or unhappy, in the hope that it is going to make a difference for us. We all know the sensation of comfort-eating, while too many 'bitter' tastes and experiences have a less desirable effect. The food and flavours of life that we put into ourselves become us, our Rasa, our essence. The supermarkets and food industry play on this, particularly in the promotion of the addictive sweet and salt tastes.

While Ayurveda identifies six tastes, Traditional Chinese Medicine identifies only five: sweet, sour, salt, pungent and bitter. They have left out the astringent taste, which is possibly experienced more as a sensation on the tongue. From the Japanese point of view, we also hear about the taste *Umami*, identified as a pleasant savoury taste – a brothy, meaty taste with a high level of glutamates. It can be found in old hard cheese, miso, mushrooms, soy sauce, kimchi, green tea, marmite and tomatoes.

Very few foods will have only one taste but it is important to work with the primary taste or tastes.

These may change according to where the food has come from, how it has been produced and how fresh and ripe it is. For example, an apple may taste sweet or sour depending on the variety selected and the climate. Garlic contains all tastes except salt.

Rasa and the Doshas

Each of the six tastes has a predominance of two of the five Pancha Maha Bhutas (elements) and therefore has an effect on the Doshas, as detailed in the table below:

Rasa (taste)	**Pancha Maha Bhutas (elements)**	**Effect on Dosha**
Sweet – *Madhura*	Earth and Water	⇑ K ⇓ VP
Sour – *Amla*	Earth and Fire	⇑ PK ⇓ V
Salt – *Lavana*	Water and Fire	⇑ PK ⇓ V
Pungent – *Katu*	Air and Fire	⇑ PV ⇓ K
Bitter – *Tikta*	Air and Ether	⇑ V ⇓ PK
Astringent – *Kasaya*	Earth and Air	⇑ V ⇓ PK

Table 4.1 Rasa and its effect on the Doshas

Vata is made up of ether and air, Pitta is made up of fire and water, and Kapha is made up of earth and water. Using the rule of 'like increases like and opposites reduce', we can identify which tastes will increase a Dosha and which tastes will reduce and balance a Dosha.

Sweet taste refers to the neutral, nourishing, natural tastes of proteins, fats and carbohydrates rather than those of highly processed sugar or sweet treats. This neutral-sweet taste is made up of the elements of earth and water, which are the same elements as Kapha Dosha. Using the rule 'like increases like', the sweet taste is going to increase and aggravate Kapha. Conversely, 'opposites reduce', so it is going to reduce Vata (as it does not contain these elements) and secondarily Pitta (which contains water but not earth).

Sour taste is made up of earth and fire. Kapha Dosha contains the earth element and Pitta Dosha the fire element so, using the rule 'like increases like', both these Doshas are increased by the sour taste. Vata contains neither of these elements and therefore sour will reduce and balance Vata Dosha.

Salt taste is made up of fire and water. Pitta is made up of fire and water and Kapha contains the water element: therefore, the salt taste increases both Pitta and Kapha Dosha. Vata contains neither the fire nor the water element and therefore salt will reduce and balance Vata Dosha.

Pungent taste is made up of fire and air. Pitta contains the fire element and Vata the air element: therefore, the pungent taste increases both Pitta and Vata. Kapha contains neither fire nor air elements and therefore pungent will reduce and balance Kapha Dosha.

Bitter taste is made up of air and ether, increasing Vata (air and ether) but reducing Pitta and Kapha, which contain neither of these elements.

Astringent taste is made up of earth and air, increasing Vata (air) but reducing Pitta, which contains neither of these elements. In small amounts the astringent taste will reduce Kapha because of the air element (Kapha has no air element), but in large amounts can increase Kapha because of the earth element (Kapha contains the earth element).

Sweet taste – Madhura

The sweet taste is heavy, cooling and oily in nature. The word *Madhura* in Sanskrit, which translates as 'sweet', is much more neutral than the way we normally understand it and does not include the very sweet taste found in sugar, sweets and fizzy drinks that are so unbalancing. Sweet is the first taste we experience, in a mother's milk; it is comforting, soothing and slightly analgesic, and we naturally develop a preference for this taste. It is building and strengthening to all body tissues, harmonises the mind and promotes a sense of contentment. However, in excess it can lead to obesity and type two diabetes. The majority of our diet is made up of the sweet taste, which includes fats, proteins and carbohydrates that give nourishment and energy. If you are mainly Pitta or Vata Dosha your diet should include about 70% of the sweet taste, whereas Kapha needs a little less.

Madhura sweet foods:

- carbohydrates – grains
- fats and oils
- protein – meat, fish, dairy products
- sweet fruit
- sweet vegetables – particularly root vegetables
- nuts and seeds
- honey and maple syrup
- unrefined sugar cane.

Sour taste – Amla

The sour taste is light, heating and oily in nature. When used in moderation, it is refreshing, stimulates the appetite, improves digestion, energises the body and awakens the mind and the senses. After the sweet taste, sour is the next major food group in our British diet. Our diet should include one to two servings of sour-tasting food, or smaller quantities as side dishes or added to cooking. Pitta Dosha can be very aggravated by eating too much of the heating sour taste which can lead to acid indigestion, itching and inflamed skin. In Northern Europe they often eat more of the sour taste where traditionally fermentation is used to preserve food to eat in the cold winter months when it is more difficult to grow fresh foods.

Sour foods:

- fermented foods – kimchi
- alcohol
- sour fruit – lemon, lime, grapefruit, sour cherry, rhubarb
- tomatoes
- pickled foods
- yoghurt
- vinegar – salad dressing
- tamari and soy sauce
- salad dressings
- bread (yeasted)
- hard cheeses.

Salt taste – Lavana

The salt taste is heating, heavy and oily in nature. When taken in moderation, it gives energy and maintains our water electrolyte balance. It enhances the flavour of our food, but in excess can overpower all other tastes. Daily intake should be about 2–6 grams (½ to 1 teaspoon) a day (NHS.UK). Like the sweet taste, it is essential for our survival and can be addictive; most of us eat too much salt, particularly as it is added to processed foods. Eating too much salt can result in high blood pressure, water retention and skin problems.

As well as salt being used in cooking and as a condiment at the dining table, it is naturally present in many foods through sea water and small amounts in the soil.

Ayurveda recommends rock salt, especially Himalayan salt as it is lighter and dryer than sea salt. Sea salt is more heating and for that reason may aggravate Pitta more. Avoid highly processed table salt.

Salt foods:

- fish from the sea
- seaweed, kelp
- soy and Worcestershire sauce
- salt – rock salt or sea salt
- parmesan cheese
- anchovies
- capers
- miso
- celery.

Pungent taste – Katu

This taste is light, drying and heating in action and is the most stimulating and heating of the tastes. It promotes and improves digestion. Used in excess it can create a burning sensation, thirst, diarrhoea, nausea and infertility.

Kapha benefits from having some of the pungent taste daily as it wakes up and stimulates the digestive system. This can be added through pungent spices, onions and garlic in cooking or as a tea infusion. However, it should be used in much smaller quantities for Vata and Pitta. In Britain we eat more of the mild pungent tastes like onions, garlic, parsley and rosemary that are grown locally. Too many heating pungent spices can feel fiery and overpowering unless you are used to eating them.

Pungent foods:

- pungent spices – cardamom, cayenne, chillies, cinnamon, cloves, coriander, cumin, mustard, oregano, parsley, black pepper, peppermint, rosemary, sage, star anise, tarragon, thyme, turmeric (pungent, bitter astringent)
- onions (sweet and pungent)
- garlic (all tastes except salt)
- radishes
- coffee (pungent and bitter)
- miso (pungent, sour and salt).

Bitter taste – Tikta

The bitter taste is cool, light and dry in nature. The bitter taste promotes all the other five tastes and reduces cravings. We are naturally wary of the bitter taste as it can be an indication of poisonous plants. By observing the eating habits of animals our ancestors learnt that, if they didn't kill you, many bitter-tasting foods and herbs eaten in small quantities could be good for you. It is worth creating a taste for bitter if you are a Pitta or Kapha type, so a portion of dark leafy greens every day helps to balance these two Doshas, but for Vata you need less. The bitter taste is cleansing, good for the blood and weight loss. However, an overuse of this taste can lead to coldness and stiffness in the body, and it can aggravate Vata Dosha.

Bitter foods:

- bitter vegetables (dark leafy greens) – some cruciferous vegetables, e.g., Brussels sprouts, kale, cabbage and chicory
- bitter herbs – dandelion greens, turmeric (bitter, pungent, astringent)
- bitter fruit – cranberries
- some drinks – coffee, green tea
- dark chocolate.

Astringent taste – Kasaya

The astringent taste is cooling, dry and heavy in nature. If you don't recognise this taste, you can experience it as a sensation of puckering, roughness and drying in the mouth as when you eat an unripe green banana. As with the bitter taste, it is worth cultivating a taste for astringent if you are a Pitta or Kapha type. A daily small portion of Legumes (pulses and beans) or an astringent vegetable balances these two Doshas and supports digestion, but for Vata you want less as the dryness can aggravate Vata and lead to constipation.

Many Ayurveda cookbooks include a lot of recipes using Legumes (pulses and beans), which are astringent but can often be too drying for Vata if they are consumed in large quantities.

Astringent foods:

- some fruits and berries – pomegranates and cranberries have some astringent quality
- some vegetables – asparagus, broccoli, celery
- beverages – tea, coffee
- beans and legumes – adzuki beans, broad beans, chickpeas, kidney beans, mung beans, butter beans, lentils, soya beans
- anything that is green produces some astringency from the chlorophyll – this might be a secondary taste.

Effect of tastes on Doshas

Using the information on Doshas and Rasa (taste) we can now start to build up a picture of which tastes and foods are best for each Dosha. In addition to the Pancha Maha Bhutas, the elements of ether, air, fire, water and earth, the Doshas and Rasa (tastes) can be identified by the Gunas – the qualities that describe everything in nature. This detail underpins why some tastes increase Dosha and others decrease Doshas.

Doshas can be identified by their Gunas:

- Vata is dry, light and cold
- Pitta is slightly oily, hot and light
- Kapha is oily, cool and heavy.

Rasas (taste) can be identified by these same Gunas:

- Sweet is heavy, cooling and oily
- Sour is light, heating and oily
- Salt is heavy, heating and oily
- Pungent is light, heating and drying
- Bitter is light, cool and drying
- Astringent is heavy, cool and drying.

Using the principle of 'like increases like and opposites reduce', we can identify the effect of taste on Dosha:

Dosha	**Increases Dosha** *Eat less*	**Decreases Dosha** *Eat more*
Vata	Pungent, bitter, astringent	Sweet, sour, salt
Pitta	Sour, salt, pungent	Sweet, bitter, astringent
Kapha	Sweet, sour, salt	Pungent, bitter, astringent

Table 4.2 Effect of taste on Doshas

Vipaka – Post-digestive taste

According to Ayurveda, secondary digestion in the liver by digestive enzymes modifies some tastes. This helps us to understand what effect food will have on the body over a longer period of time, rather than just supplying the immediate taste.

After food has been assimilated – generally six to eight hours – a post-digestive 'taste' emerges. The six tastes (sweet, sour, salt, pungent, bitter and astringent) are consolidated, leaving three post-digestive tastes (*Vipaka*) that remain:

Rasa	**Vipaka**	**Effect on Dosha**
Sweet	Sweet	Increase Kapha
Salt	Sweet	Increase Pitta/ Kapha
Sour	Sour	Increase Pitta/ Kapha
Pungent	Pungent	Increase Vata/ Pitta
Bitter	Pungent	Increase Vata
Astringent	Pungent	Increase Vata/ Pitta

Table 4.3 Vipaka effect on Dosha

5. Gunas and Food

The Gunas are ten pairs of attributes or qualities that can be used to describe the characteristics of everything in nature. We use these attributes to describe the Doshas and to describe food. This information gives us a template to understand which foods support a Dosha and which create imbalance because of their matching Gunas. Each pair of opposites works on a continuum: for example, between very cold and very hot there is cool and warm.

The Gunas that have the most effect on the Doshas and on diet are:

- hot and cold
- heavy and light
- oily/wet and dry.

We use these Gunas to evaluate the effect that foods will have on the body.

In cooking we refer to the texture of food, the properties of food that are sensed in the mouth; we use descriptive words like 'smooth', 'lumpy', 'crumbly' and 'creamy'. This is much more about likes and dislikes, memory and association, as well as being used in recipe instructions: for example, we talk of lumpy custard or the velvety smooth, rich texture of a chocolate mousse; factors that affect our perception of food.

However, the twenty Gunas in Ayurveda come from the Maha Gunas of Sattva, Rajas and Tamas. This helps us to observe in an objective and logical way how these Gunas affect us and to be more selective over which foods to eat.

Guna	Effect on Dosha
Hot/warm	↑P ↓VK
Cold/cool	↑VK ↓P
Heavy	↑K ↓VP
Light	↑VP ↓K
Oily/wet	↑PK ↓V
Dry	↑V ↓PK

Table 5.1 Gunas and their effect on Dosha

Hot and cold

Heating	Pungent	Sour	Salty
Cooling	Bitter	Astringent	Sweet

All food has either heating or cooling properties, although the strength of this can change. For instance, carrots are warming and almost neutral, whereas chilli and cayenne pepper are extremely heating.

Heating foods

Heating foods will dilate the channels (*Srotamsi*) of the body – one of the most obvious effects being an increased pulse rate and sweating after eating a hot curry. Heating foods can reduce mucus and phlegm and improve Agni, our digestive capacity.

Hot reduces Vata and Kapha and increases Pitta.

A small number of foods are extremely heating, including alcohol, chilli peppers, cayenne pepper, mustard, horseradish and dry ginger. Onions and garlic are also classified as heating; however, this does vary slightly depending on the variety grown, the climate and whether they are eaten raw or cooked.

There is a much larger range of foods that are described as warming or mildly heating, including avocados, carrots, leeks, pumpkins, tomatoes, oats, quinoa, rye, lentils, almonds, goat's milk, yoghurt, fish, meat, eggs, honey, coffee, salt, vinegar, cumin, rosemary, sage, thyme and turmeric. These foods will aggravate Pitta when eaten in excess.

Cooling foods

Cooling foods can create congestion or stagnation and slow the digestive system. This can be seen with dairy products, which are cooling, heavy and moist and can create catarrh and phlegm. On the other hand, the effect of cooling food is beneficial for Pitta and reduces inflammation and general heat in the body.

Cool reduces Pitta and increases Vata and Kapha.

Iced cold drinks and food including ice cream will shock and suppress digestion by affecting the digestive fire. In the same way that we are shocked and shiver if we dive into really cold water, the body goes into shock when we eat and drink really cold foods. This results in the digestive fire being extinguished and the system shutting down.

There is a large range of foods that are described as cooling, including apples, blueberries, lemons, raspberries, strawberries, asparagus, broccoli, Brussels sprouts, cabbage, celery, lettuce, olives, potatoes, muesli, basmati rice, wheat (but not fermented bread), mung beans, kidney beans, dhal, adzuki beans, soy products, butter, cow's milk, hard cow's cheese, ghee, milk and maple syrup.

Heavy and light

Heavy foods

Heavy foods can be difficult to digest, can decrease our Agni (digestive fire) and are mostly found in the earth element and secondarily in water. They are nourishing and grounding but eaten in excess can create weight gain and dullness.

Heavy reduces Vata and Pitta (slightly) and increases Kapha.

Heavy foods include red meat, fish, fried foods, dairy, bananas, avocados, dates, figs, aubergines, mushrooms, soybeans, hard cheese and nuts. Red meat is regarded as the heaviest and most difficult food to digest.

Most root vegetables are categorised as heavy, which is why a root vegetable soup in winter is beneficial for Vata and will give heaviness and a grounding effect. Grains including oats, pasta, brown rice and wheat are considered heavy, as they contain significant amounts of the earth element that builds tissue and provides fibre to the body.

Light foods

Light foods bring lightness to the body. When eaten in excess they deplete body tissues and result in weight loss. They clear the channels of the body, are easy to digest, and increase Agni.

Light reduces Kapha and increases Vata and Pitta (slightly).

Lighter foods include many fruits, and include apples, berries, raisins, leafy vegetables, Brussels sprouts, spinach, lettuce, salads, sprouted seeds, popcorn, amaranth, barley, millet, basmati rice, red lentils, mung beans, white chicken meat, cardamom, cinnamon, ginger and turmeric.

Wet and dry

Moist foods

The moist Guna is more than just clear, wet water; it has a slightly oily or unctuous quality to it, as in blood plasma or olive oil. Wet/oily moistens and lubricates, creating smoothness, flexibility and softness.

Oily/wet reduces Vata and increases Kapha and Pitta.

Moist foods include berries, avocados, ghee, oils and fats, dairy, cheese, eggs, oily fish, nuts, nut butter and seeds, as well as dishes such as soup, dhal and stew, but not plain water.

Dry foods

Dry foods can create dehydration, dry skin and constipation.

Dry reduces Pitta and Kapha (slightly) and increases Vata.

Drying foods include dry grains and cereal, millet, oats, beans and pulses, chickpeas, mung beans, toast, dried fruits, dark leafy greens, broccoli, kale, mushrooms, potatoes, spinach, corn, artichokes, popcorn, black pepper and turmeric. Many of these foods require moisture to make them edible and to counteract their extreme dryness.

Gunas and Food

Life, however, is never simple. Although all foods will be either heating or cooling in varying degrees, they will also have other attributes that must also be taken into consideration when planning the correct foods for specific Doshas.

Food	Taste	Gunas	Action on Dosha
Sweet potato	Sweet	Cooling, soft, heavy	Increase Kapha
White potato	Astringent	Cooling, dry, light, rough	Increase Vata
Raw carrot	Astringent	Warming, hard, rough, heavy	Increase Vata & Pitta
Cooked carrot	Sweet	Warming, light, soft	Increase Pitta in excess

Table 5.2. Examples of Gunas and food

6. Sattva, Rajas and Tamas in Food

In Ayurveda the effect of eating different types of food will influence our mental balance and behaviour as well our physical health and wellbeing. Foods express the Gunas of Sattva, Rajas and Tamas. In our efforts to attain a Sattvic or balanced state of mind we want to eat a diet that is predominant in the Sattvic Guna.

A Sattvic diet is mainly made up of organic fresh fruit and vegetables, grains, basmati rice, mung beans, fresh dairy products and ghee. Foods that promote Sattva are pure and balancing, fresh and as natural as possible; they bring purity, calm, joy and increased energy.

Rajasic foods include most spices, some beans, potatoes, tomatoes and sour fruit. From the perspective of Ayuverda we should seek to reduce our use of Rajasic foods; although a cup of coffee might get you going in the morning, to be dependent on it to get through the day can make you jumpy, restless, angry and controlling, which are all Rajasic-type emotions.

Tamasic foods include fermented, stale, left-over and over-ripe foods, mushrooms, eggs and meat.

Foods that promote Tamas are generally impure or dead (with no Prana or vitality), which creates heaviness, lethargy, depression and ill health. Reheated food, microwaved food, fried food, barbequed food, food with preservative, takeaways and ready prepared meals are all considered to be Tamasic.

The tables that follow identify food as Sattvic, Rajasic or Tamasic and enable us to look at food from a slightly different perspective, that of how food affects our mental health. There is a degree of subjectivity attached that can vary according to different schools of Ayurveda teaching. As always, it is important to observe the effect of the food we eat.

Foods	**Sattvic**
Fruit	Most fresh seasonal fruit
Vegetables	Most fresh seasonal vegetables
Grains	Most grains
Beans/ lentils	Mung and adzuki beans, red lentils, fresh beans
Dairy	Raw, organic cow's milk, ghee
Nuts and seeds	All fresh nuts and seeds
Culinary spices	Most fresh culinary herbs and spices
Sweeteners	Fresh sugarcane juice, jaggery, raw sugar, raw honey (if bees are not harmed), maple syrup
Beverages	Herbal fruit and spicy teas, fresh fruit juice

Meat	
Eggs	

Table 6.1 Sattva and Food

Foods	**Rajasic**
Fruit	Sour fruit, bananas
Vegetables	Potatoes, tomatoes, peppers, aubergines, chillies, pickles, onions, garlic, leeks
Grains	
Beans/ lentils	Most dried and tinned legumes and lentils, including soya
Dairy	**Butter, cottage cheese, cream, kefir, sour cream, cottage cheese, products from goats or sheep
Nuts and seeds	
Culinary spices	Chilli, cayenne and black pepper
Sweeteners	Processed sugar, cooked honey, dark chocolate
Beverages	Coffee, black and green tea (caffeine), alcohol
Meat	
Eggs	

Table 6.2 Rajas and Food

Foods	**Tamasic**
Fruit	
Vegetables	Mushrooms, garlic, onions
Grains	Modern processed wheat

Beans/ lentils	Salted peanuts
Dairy	All heat-treated dairy, e.g. pasteurised, homogenised, ice cream, hard aged cheese, margarine
Nuts and seeds	Rancid nuts
Culinary spices	Nutmeg
Sweeteners	Artificial sweeteners, soft drinks, very sweet-tasting foods
Beverages	Alcohol (larger quantities)
Meat	All meat and fish*
Eggs	Eggs*

Table 6.3 Tamas and Food

*This is why spiritual diets often do not contain meat, fish or eggs.

**There are degrees of variation – a hard cheddar cheese could be considered more Rajasic and heating than cottage cheese.

7. Food Groups

Sourcing of food

Before we get into a detailed look at food, it is important to consider where food is sourced from and how it is produced. Over the last fifty years, as a nation we have produced more food for less money, and we spend a lower percentage of our income on food. In the 1940s about a third of average household income was spent on food, compared with 14% nowadays. This created an agricultural drive to produce and import food more cheaply, which has had a consequential negative affect on food quality, our health, and our world. Proportionately, we spend less money on food in the UK than most other countries around the world.

Ayurveda originated at a time when food was organic, grown locally and eaten fresh. As a result, it was full of Prana and connected to the local environment, seasons and nature, which is how we have evolved to eat.

It is really worth evaluating the quality of the food you are purchasing and consuming – after all, we are what we eat. So, if we consume a diet with little or no nutritional goodness or Prana then over time our physical and mental health will reflect this.

It is recommended to eat the best-quality food that you can afford: ideally fresh, organic and locally produced, free from pesticides, fungicides, fertilisers, antibiotics and other chemicals. It is also advisable to avoid processed foods, especially ready meals and ultra-processed foods, which lack freshness and Prana and contain added ingredients and chemicals that our bodies don't recognise or know what to do with.

As this book focuses on Ayurveda, I have only briefly touched on food from a modern nutritional perspective. Scientific research can deepen our understanding of how to make good food choices; for example, many of our popular grocery items such as iceberg lettuce and Golden Delicious apples are poorer choices when compared with traditional heritage varieties that have more nutrients in them. Additionally, some medication has contraindications with specific food and herbs; for example, people taking MAOI (monoamine oxidase inhibitor) drugs used to treat depression should avoid foods that are high in tyramine, which is found in broad beans, aged cheese, cured meat, yeast extract and beer. If you are taking medication, it is always worth checking the 'small print' for these finer details.

We have an epidemic of chronic ill health, including gut inflammation, heart disease, diabetes, dementia, cancer, high blood pressure, obesity and autoimmune disorders. There is an increasing body of scientific research that clearly demonstrates a correlation between the state of our diet and our health. As we have already identified, according to Ayurveda all disease begins with Ama.

Simple guidance includes: 'Don't eat anything your (great) grandmother wouldn't have recognised as food' and 'Don't buy anything with more than five ingredients'.

Fruit

Generally, fruit is light, refreshing, cooling, cleansing and Sattvic in nature.

Ayurveda recommends eating locally produced fruit when it is in season, ideally organic; when this is not possible, washing and peeling fruit helps. We are often spoilt for choice in supermarkets with fruit flown in from around the world when it is out of season here in the UK. However, most soft fruits and berries ripen in the summer heat and apples and pears ripen in early autumn when they are at their best. Generally, we want to eat less fruit in the cold winter months.

A small amount of fruit is good for all of us, though fruit is best for Pitta and then Vata Dosha, with Kapha Dosha needing less fruit. Pitta Dosha is best with sweet fruit rather than sour-tasting fruits that can cause Dosha aggravation; this is particularly so for grapefruits and lemons. Vata Dosha can eat sweet- and sour-tasting fruit, although fruit can cause bloating and gas when digestion is sensitive. Cooking fruit before eating it can be a good idea, especially for Vata Dosha and in the winter months. Stewed fruit benefits from adding a few sweet digestive spices: cinnamon, ginger, cardamom and cloves rather than sugar. Small quantities of dried fruit, with its reduced water content, are good for Kapha but should be avoided by Vata.

It is suggested that fruit is best eaten on its own or at the beginning of the meal and not mixed with other food ingredients. Fruit is digested quickly and easily and, if eaten after something heavy such as meat, can ferment while the meat is being digested and cause wind and bloating. Whatever is eaten first is digested first. However, not all modern science agrees with this, identifying that there are times when it could be beneficial to eat fruit with protein and fat in order to slow down the digestion of the fruit and reduce the impact on blood sugar levels.

Fruit makes a good choice for breakfast or as a snack. Fruit juice and smoothies should be used with caution, owing to their concentrated sweetness and lack of fibre. It is better to make your own, using no more than three fresh fruits and no extras, rather than buying it ready prepared; that way you know what's in it. Melons are often difficult to digest and should only be eaten on their own.

Some fruits are well known for their medicinal benefits, including prunes, figs and dates as laxatives and fresh cranberries (with no added sugar) to help prevent urinary tract infections. Grapefruit, in particular, has an adverse interaction with many medications, including statins and drugs to treat high blood pressure, and should therefore be avoided.

Vegetables

Vegetables are excellent for all Doshas. They should form a major part of our daily diet and be eaten in abundance – including nourishing, earthy root vegetables and green, leafy vegetables that are full of nutrients and fibre. It is ideally best to eat a wide variety of locally grown organic vegetables in season.

Vegetables mix with all other foods (except fruit), especially grains. Eat the rainbow; choose vegetables that have a wide variety of colours when they are available. The different coloured vegetables each contain powerful plant chemicals that are good for our health.

Fungi and mushrooms are not generally covered in Ayurveda because they are considered to be Tamasic. But we should not overlook them, as they are a useful alternative to meat; modern research is showing that they have many health benefits. They are sweet, astringent and cooling but are hard to digest and increase Vata.

- Vata Dosha can eat most vegetables, especially sweet nutritious root vegetables, including sweet potatoes, carrots and beetroot that should be well cooked. Avocados and squash are also good for Vata. Vata are advised to limit eating raw vegetables, including onions and salad, owing to their cold, dry, light Gunas, especially in the cold winter months. Vegetables from the cabbage family including cauliflower, Brussels sprouts, kale, broccoli and cabbage are astringent in taste and can result in gas and bloating for Vata types if eaten in excess.

- Pitta Dosha can eat most vegetables, including some raw vegetables and salad, due to their cooling nature. The exceptions are heating pungent vegetables such as raw onions, radishes, garlic and watercress. Pitta types are often sensitive to vegetables from the Solanaceae family, which consists of tomatoes, potatoes, aubergines, peppers and chillies. Avocados are heavy and unctuous and should be eaten only in moderation.

- Kapha Dosha do well with leafy green vegetables, including cabbage, broccoli, celery and Brussels sprouts. They benefit from eating astringent, pungent and bitter-tasting vegetables, including cauliflower, Swiss chard, garlic, green beans, kale, leeks, onions, peas, pumpkins and spinach. They are advised to limit sweet potatoes, summer squashes and avocados, which are sweet and heavy, and raw vegetables.

The Five a Day Campaign, advocated by the World Health Organization and the UK NHS, recommends eating five portions of fruit and vegetables a day, which has been proven to lower the risk of serious health problems and mortality. More recent gut health experts are now taking this a stage further and adding the recommendation to eat at least thirty different plant-based foods a week.

Grains

The grains that suit us depend on our Sātmya – where we were born and what we can tolerate. Each civilisation has thrived on a particular grain: rice in Asia, wheat in America and Europe, corn in Latin America, rye in Scandinavia.

Fresh whole grains are generally sweet in taste, neutral in energy, nourishing and Sattvic. They contain larger amounts of the earth element, which is necessary to build tissues and provides fibre that gives bulk to the stool (faeces). We have learnt to transform grains by grinding and cooking to make them easier to digest, and in Ayurveda they are consumed along with spices. Steamed whole grains are very balanced and the easiest form of grain to digest. They should form an important part of our diet, especially for Vata and Pitta Dosha.

Many people are familiar with only a few of the available grains – probably wheat, rice and oats.

However, there are many other grains that are worth trying: rye bread, spelt bread, barley added to soups and stews, quinoa as an alternative to rice, amaranth, buckwheat and millet. Each of these grains has its own Gunas (qualities). They are fairly neutral in energy, making then suitable for all Doshas. Kapha Dosha benefit from eating a smaller quantity of grains, especially wheat and oats, than do Vata and Pitta.

In the UK we have developed an over-dependence on wheat, which is often highly processed as breakfast cereal and toast for breakfast, sandwiches for lunch, and pizza and pasta dishes for supper, as well as being used in many processed foods. The wheat we eat today has been hybridised and is not the same as our ancestors ate. Consequently, many of us have difficulty digesting wheat that contains gluten, especially in bread when yeast is added. Modern bread is often made too quickly without leaving the dough to rise naturally. Instead, more yeast is used, which can be very aggravating to Pitta. This can cause Ama, bloating, wind or more serious health issues such as inflammation, brain fog, intestinal permeability ('leaky gut') and coeliac disease (gluten allergy).

It is helpful to eat a wide variety of grains. The Coeliac Society has useful information on gluten-free grains and flours, including how to blend different flours for various recipes. Maize, rice, potato, tapioca and cornflour are some of the more common gluten-free flours available. It makes no sense to choose a highly processed wheat flour that has had the gluten removed and now lacks any vitality. Supermarkets and health food shops sell gluten-free flour made from a blend of naturally gluten-free grains. Many people find traditionally made sourdough bread easier to digest than yeasted bread as it has no added yeast. Most flatbreads such as Indian chapatis do not include yeast and can be made from a variety of flours, including gram flour, which is made from chickpeas. (Coeliac Society - *See 'Other links' in the Bibliography.*)

As Ayurveda originates from India, rice is often the first grain of choice in Ayurveda cookery books. You need to use your own judgement as to whether you can easily digest rice and how often you choose to eat it. Basmati rice suits all three Doshas and is considered easier to digest; brown rice and wild rice are good for Vata Dosha but slightly unbalancing for Pitta and Kapha Dosha. Avoid bleached, refined white rice.

Legumes – pulses and beans

Pulses are the dried seeds of legumes and include mung beans, adzuki beans, chickpeas, black beans, lima beans, kidney beans, haricot beans, lentils and soya beans. Soya is used in many ways including in tofu, milk, edamame and fermented miso, tempeh and soya sauce. Legumes are a staple food in many cuisines across the world, including the UK up until the Middle Ages when meat and dairy produce became more affordable to most of the population. Perhaps the most popular way of eating beans in the UK is as tinned baked beans in a sweet tomato sauce, of which we consume two million cans every day.

Pulses and beans are a versatile form of nutrition. They are high in protein but can be astringent, drying and hard to digest, especially for Vata Dosha, causing gas and constipation. Most beans are Rajasic and can have an irritant effect on the body and mind. Unless you can easily digest pulses and beans, it is suggested that you eat them no more than once or twice a week for Vata Dosha, two to three times a week for Pitta Dosha and three to four times a week for Kapha Dosha.

Mung and adzuki beans are considered easier to digest, especially for Vata and Pitta Dosha, and lentils are another good choice for Kapha Dosha. Generally, the bigger the bean the harder they are to digest. Spices, especially asafoetida, can be added to them in the cooking process to counteract the difficulty of digestion.

Peanuts also belong to the legume family. Peanuts are a common allergy-causing food. A severe allergic reaction can sometimes result in anaphylaxis, causing the body to go into shock.

Legumes are high in compounds called lectins (proteins that are bound to carbohydrates). In high concentrations these can be difficult to digest and when eaten in excess can damage the gut wall and cause an upset stomach. Before cooking, many dried beans require soaking and rinsing well; they should then be boiled well (skimming any foam off the top) and cooked until they are very soft. Soaking and cooking dried legumes at a high temperature deactivates most lectins, making them safe to eat and more easily digestible. Buying tinned beans is often easier than starting with dried if you don't eat beans that often.

Nuts and seeds

Most fresh nuts and seeds are slightly sweet, warming and highly nutritious, but are also heavy, oily and hard to digest. They are a good source of vegetable protein and fat and are considered to be Sattvic in nature. They decrease Vata but increase both Kapha and Pitta. They should be used in very small amounts, especially for Pitta and Kapha. Coconut is one of the few nuts that are cooling and therefore beneficial for Pitta.

Nuts grown in England include hazelnut, chestnut and walnut; nuts grown in Europe include almonds, pistachios, pine nuts and pecan nuts. Seeds include flax seeds, sunflower seeds and pumpkin seeds. Eat a variety of different nuts for different snacks and meals.

The whole fresh nut is difficult to digest – but nuts don't have to be eaten whole! They can be toasted gently, ground, made into a nut butter, used as nut oils or made into gomasio (sesame salt). The key is to take small amounts regularly: one small handful a day for Vata and Pitta, while Kapha should have them only from time to time, as otherwise they can reduce and slow Agni (digestive fire).

It is best to buy fresh organic nuts in their natural state (still in their shells) where possible and without added salt to ensure that they are not stale or rancid.

Dairy

Traditional Ayurveda saw milk as Sattvic and a health-giving food. Modern farming methods and pasteurisation often compromises the goodness of milk making it Tamasic, especially with the widespread use of antibiotics. Therefore, it is recommended to use organic milk and dairy produce. If you choose to use raw milk always buy from a reputable source and boil the milk to kill any bacteria present in it.

Milk and most dairy products are sweet, cooling and nourishing. They are beneficial for Vata and Pitta in small amounts but is not recommended for Kapha. They are good for children, for the elderly and during convalescence as good sources of protein and fats. Goat's milk is more astringent and warming, making it slightly better for Kapha.

Milk is best consumed warm as cold milk can be hard to digest and forms Ama. The addition of spices such as cardamom, cinnamon ginger and clove improves the digestion of milk, especially for Vata Dosha.

Fermenting milk to produce yoghurt, kefir, sour cream or cheese makes it more heating and aggravating for Pitta Dosha. Pitta Dosha do better with soft, fresh cheese such as cottage cheese rather than a hard or blue cheese. Some fermented dairy products, including yoghurt and kefir, are probiotics and good for gut health; however, you need only a small amount.

Ghee or clarified butter is highly valued in Ayurveda. It is suitable for all three Doshas, has many health benefits, is good for digestion and has a long storage life. It is a good fat to cook with, as it withstands the heating process to 230 °C.

The use of low-fat processed dairy produce and milks is not recommended; it is better to use full-fat milk and then dilute it with water. Ice cream is ice-cold and should be kept for an occasional treat, especially for Vata and Kapha.

Dairy – alternative non-dairy products

A number of different non-dairy milks are now available.

You can choose to make your own non-dairy milk by soaking, grinding and blending your own chosen alternative – for example, organic almond nuts, soya beans or oats – with filtered water either in a blender or in a plant-milk-maker machine. This avoids it being highly processed through adding sugar and preservatives.

Almond milk is good for Vata as it is warming, unctuous and heavy; soya milk is a good milk for Pitta as it is sweet and cooling.

Oils and fats

We all benefit from a small amount of fats and oils in our diet. It gives the body energy, protects the organs, supports cell growth, helps the body absorb nutrients, and is essential for brain function.

There is much confusion relating to fats and oils but there is a growing body of evidence suggesting that reducing saturated fats in the diet has no significantly beneficial effect on cardiovascular health. The fats to avoid are hydrogenated or trans-fats that are found in margarine and processed food. Many countries have banned trans-fats, but they are still permitted in the UK and the USA.

Culinary vegetable oils are made from nuts and seeds. A wide choice is available, including almond, coconut, olive, sesame, sunflower, walnut and mustard oil. Fresh cold-pressed, unrefined, quality raw vegetable oils are Sattvic, mostly sweet and bland in taste, and slightly warm in energy. Coconut and olive oil are both cooling and so are better for Pitta Dosha. The classic oil used in Ayurveda is sesame oil, which is a good all-round oil and particularly useful in cooking, with a smoke point of 232 °C. Olive oil is the classic oil of the Mediterranean diet; the Greeks call it 'liquid gold' because of its many health benefits.

Vata, owing to its drying attribute, needs a regular diet containing good fats and oils. Pitta is fine if consuming a moderate amount of them, whilst Kapha needs the least amount of fat.

Fish

Fish are nutritious, Tamasic, sweet in taste, warming in quality and less heavy to digest than meat.

The pollution in our seas and oceans is having a concerning effect on the quality of our fish, especially through pollutants such as mercury. Small fish such as sardines will contain less than do larger fish such as tuna. Much of the fish stock bought in supermarkets is farmed and comes from an environment where over-crowding of the fish can create a proliferation of bacteria and require the consequent use of antibiotics. Ayurveda does not advocate using shellfish. Trout is one of the easiest fish to digest.

Vata does well with oily fish such as salmon, mackerel, anchovies, sardines and herring, whereas in theory Pitta will do better with freshwater fish that are less salty and heating than are seawater fish. However, oily fish is an excellent source of the polyunsaturated fatty acid Omega 3 which is linked to many health benefits for all of us.

Meat

Generally, meat is not recommended in Ayurveda, which does however acknowledge that meat is nourishing and uses it as a broth or soup for people who are convalescing or need building up. It is heavy, Tamasic, difficult to digest unless taken as a soup, and can create Ama. It is balancing for Vata but can aggravate Pitta and Kapha. Organic chicken from a reputable source is lighter and easier to digest than red meat for all three Doshas if you wish to include a little meat in your diet.

Sweeteners

From birth we are attracted to the sweet taste, starting with mother's milk to ensure that we get enough nourishment. As a nation we consume too much sugar and sweeteners – nearly three times the daily recommendations of 30g a day (UK NHS) – and it is now considered to be a significant cause of today's chronic health issues. However, even despite the sugar tax in the UK it is a relatively cheap commodity.

Sugar comes from a wide variety of plants, including sugar cane, sugar beets, coconut and oil palm. These plants are then processed to produce sugar. These chemically refined processed sugars and artificially-made sweeteners arguably have no nutritional value and have been described as 'white poison'. It is best to avoid them.

Artificial sweeteners hailed by the diet industry as having no calories were believed to have no effect on the body. However, according to modern research this is far from the case, and they are thought to be just as harmful, if not more so, than sugar. As advised by the World Health Organization, it is best to avoid them. (Reference: bbcgoodfood.com *Are sweeteners bad for you?* by Jo Williams, June 2023.)

Sugars and sweeteners have many names, including granulated sugar, caster sugar, raw sugar, sugar syrup, xylitol, saccharin, sucralose and aspartame. They are used extensively in processed foods as well as in patisserie, sweet treats, confectionery and fizzy drinks.

Natural raw organic uncooked honey and raw non-refined sugars such as grade-A maple sugar and jaggery, commonly used in India, are considered to be the healthier option but they should not be heated or used in cooking. Ayurveda views honey as a good source of sweetness; it is Sattvic and warming with a sweet, astringent and pungent taste. It is good for Vata and Kapha and aggravates Pitta only if taken in large quantities and in the summer months.

Generally, natural sweet-tasting foods decrease Pitta and Vata and increase Kapha. The exceptions are raw honey and maple syrup, which can be used for Kapha in moderation. Sweeteners should be treated as a luxury and used only in small amounts.

Culinary herbs and spices

Herbs have been used all around the world for their medicinal properties since ancient times. Cooking with herbs and spices is a wonderful way of adding flavour, as well as taking advantage of their digestive and health-giving properties. Herbal teas and infusions are another good way of benefiting from nature's bounty. Where possible, when buying fresh or dried herbs and spices choose organic and ensure that their natural properties have not been removed.

When referring to herbs in cooking, we usually mean the leaves of a plant such as rosemary or parsley. Spices usually come from the non-leafy part of the plant: the root, bark, berries, flowers and seeds. Herbs and spices cover an array of flavours from very mild to very strong, from sweet to bitter. Northern Europe tends to grow milder herbs that match the milder climate. Stronger, pungent hot spices come from countries with more dramatic hot climates, such as India and South America. Often, we only need a pinch of a spice or herb to enhance the flavour of a dish and aid digestion.

Spices are best for Kapha and Vata; Pitta is better with sweet cooling herbs rather than pungent heating spices.

A word of caution when buying and using herbs and spices. It is much safer to buy herbs and herbal formulas from a reputable herbalist or Ayurveda practitioner than from the internet. Medicinal herbal formulas are traditionally used in Ayurveda to balance Doshas and treat a wide range of health concerns. These Ayurveda formulas often have to be adapted using herbs and spices that can safely be used or imported to the UK. It also ensures that the formula you buy is safe and right for you. Even culinary herbs and spices should be treated with respect and caution. For example, nutmeg is a sedative and wonderful in a milk drink to sooth the nerves, but you need only a few shavings – nutmeg is toxic, and a large dose can be lethal.

Additionally, some herbs and spices can have contrary indicators with medication, especially when taken medicinally or as food supplements. For example, turmeric has blood thinning properties so should be avoided by people taking blood thinners such as warfarin, and ginger lowers blood sugar level and should not be combined with diabetes medication except under medical supervision.

Herb	Heating/ Cooling	Vata & Kapha	Pitta
Basil	Warm	√	←
Bay leaf	Warm	√	←
Black pepper	Warm	√	X
Cinnamon	Heating	√	←
Coriander	Cooling	√	√
Cumin	Warm	√	←
Fennel	Warm	√	√
Ginger (fresh)	Heating	√	←
Nutmeg	Warm	√	←
Peppermint	Cooling	√	√
Rosemary	Warm	√	←
Sage	Warm	√	←
Tarragon	Warm	√	←
Thyme	Warm	√	←
Turmeric	Warm	√	√

Table 7.1 Common culinary herbs and spices for each Dosha

Code
√ – good to eat
←– OK in moderation
X – limit this spice

Chutneys, pickles and fermented foods

Chutneys, pickles, accompaniments and many fermented foods add a spike of flavour to a dish as well as aiding digestion, especially when they include pungent and bitter tastes. This often helps to complete the six tastes in a meal.

Both Indian and Western cuisine have naturally embraced this – a small amount of horseradish sauce as an accompaniment to beef, mint sauce with lamb, tartare sauce with fish, and mango chutney with curry.

Although it is not traditionally part of Ayurveda, you can start the meal with a small appetiser of a spoonful of sauerkraut or similar to add a little bit of fermented food into the diet. If it doesn't naturally go with your main dish, perhaps include a small green salad. A small amount of fermented food in our diet is good for our gut health and microbiome.

A common belief according to Ayurveda is that fermented food should be avoided. However, in India and in Ayurveda, plenty of fermented foods have been used over hundreds of years, such as paneer, lassi and vegetable chutneys. Many of the fermentation processes involved are short and overnight, and therefore possibly less Tamasic and less heating. Other probiotic foods include yoghurt, kefir, sauerkraut, tempeh, kimchi, miso, kombucha, sourdough bread and buttermilk.

Chutneys, pickles and fermented foods are used in small amounts, as too much can especially aggravate Vata and Pitta.

Desserts

Ayurveda does not advocate the regular use of desserts and puddings. Save desserts for special occasions or once a week at the weekend as a treat. Fruit should be eaten on its own, as a snack or at the beginning of a meal. Only eat yoghurt at lunchtime and not in the evening, as it is heavy.

However, there are times when a little bit of sweetness at the end of a meal just gives that added sense of satisfaction and completion. I suggest that a milk pudding, warm stewed fruit, fruit crumble or a dried date are healthier compromises; avoid raw fruit and desserts made using processed sugar. Another option is little sweet treats of dried fruit, nuts and/or seeds, with coconut oil to bind the ingredients into little balls, called Bliss Balls; avoid the recipes that use grain flour – you can use ground almond or coconut flour instead. These are also useful as a healthy afternoon snack or to add to a lunch box. Keep the portion sizes small. Be warned, they can become moreish but normally one (or two!) is enough!

Vegan, vegetarian or carnivore diet

This is a decision that each individual must make for themselves.

The vegetarian diet in India probably developed as a result of the Brahmin tradition and not wanting to kill animals for food. There are certainly environmental, ethical and, for some, spiritual reasons for choosing not to eat the flesh of animals.

Ayurveda has always promoted a plant-based diet. Meat-eating, however, is discussed in the classical Ayurvedic texts and is as much a part of Ayurveda as is vegetarianism. It is understood that meat is heavy and difficult to digest. Bone broth is a classic Ayurvedic dish that is easy to digest and is ideal for convalescence and gut health.

Veganism, as such, was not part of traditional Ayurveda, but obviously every type of diet can be formulated from an Ayurvedic point of view. Vegetarians and vegans should add more fresh fruit and vegetables to their diet and seek to avoid the overly processed foods that are now available in the supermarkets. If people are going to follow a vegan diet, it is important to understand how to eat a good balanced diet to get the nutrients you need, including vitamin B12, iron, zinc, calcium and essential fatty acids, as otherwise it can lead to health problems over time.

People with a predominant Vata Dosha often struggle with a vegetarian diet. They benefit from heavier and more grounding foods, whereas Kapha often fare well on a predominantly lighter vegetarian diet.

Part 3:
How to use the principles of Ayurveda in our diet

8. General Advice

Here are some general principles that will support your health and digestion. They apply to everyone. Often even simple changes can have profound results.

Eat a fresh wholefood diet. This is about eating food in its closest state to nature. These foods contain Prana, giving us vitality and health. Use foods that are good for the whole person – soul, mind and body – with the vitality of fresh fruit, vegetables and grains promoting Sattva (peace and creativity).

Use good-quality local seasonal ingredients to connect with nature and the local environment. Supermarkets offer us a wide range of ingredients from all around the world and it is easy to lose our connection to nature and our local environment. Our bodies are designed to eat food seasonally.

The freshness of food is important. Fresh, organic food has the highest Prana content. Regardless of sell-by dates, the fresher the food the more Prana and vitality it has. Nothing beats eating fruit and vegetables straight from the garden.

It's worth checking out the 'Dirty Dozen' and the 'Clean Fifteen' websites (for the twelve fruit and vegetable ingredients (which include packed salads, strawberries and apples) that have a high residue of pesticides, and the fifteen (that include avocado, cauliflower and peas) that have the lowest concentration. (*See 'Other links' in the Bibliography.*)

Avoid highly processed foods that are not in their natural state, lack Prana and contain chemical ingredients that the digestive fire, our Agni, does not understand. Sadly, we eat more processed food in the UK than any other country in the world, which is having a detrimental effect on our health.

The NOVA food classification system (reference: https://world.openfoodfacts.org/nova) identifies the degree of food processing:

1. Unprocessed or minimal processing – fruit, vegetables
2. Processed culinary ingredients – butter, sugar, salt
3. Processed food – tinned beans, smoked meat, canned fish
4. Ultra-processed foods and drinks – fizzy drinks, ready meals, margarine, sweet and savoury packaged snacks, mass-produced bread and take-away meals.

There are varying degrees of processed foods and for many food items it is about selecting our food ingredients wisely for our budget. We might use processed culinary organic maple syrup as a healthier choice to white processed sugar. When you do buy processed food, it is always worth checking the label, as some are better than others. It is advisable to avoid ultra-processed foods that are manufactured for profit rather than health – using chemicals to enhance texture, flavour and shelf life and reduce costs – and are potentially addictive, leaving us wanting more.

It is often easier and cheaper than you might think to prepare and cook your own meals, as well as being healthier. When you use fresh tasty produce, whether it's eggs in an herb omelette, spring asparagus, watercress soup or a seasonal salad, keep it simple and let the food ingredient be the star of the show.

Chew your food well, savouring each taste and feeling what it does for your body. Digestion starts in the mouth; the saliva contains enzymes needed to start the process of digesting carbohydrates, and also makes it much easier for your stomach to digest what you are sending it.

Most of us eat too fast and don't chew our food well. Slowing down and eating more mindfully will help to encourage you to chew food well before you swallow it, which is much kinder to the body as well as to the mind.

The general advice is to chew your food for about 32 bites until the food has lost its texture, although some enthusiasts say 50 bites! A bonus from this is that we often then eat less as we hear the internal 'I'm full' message, which often gets lost when we eat too fast.

Many of us would benefit from eating a little less. One tip from Ayurveda encourages us to listen for the first burp – this will tell us that we have taken in enough and should stop eating. This normally occurs when we are about 80% full, so don't overfill the stomach! Ayurveda recommends filling the stomach with 50% food and 25% liquid, leaving 25% empty to support digestion. As a rough guide, your empty stomach is the same size as your two clenched fists and stretches to hold the food you eat, so ideally you do not want to eat more than about two fistfuls or a medium-sized plate of food.

Additionally, meals should neither be excessively lingered over nor rushed; neither eating on the run nor eating a five-course banquet over several hours is good for our digestion.

Avoid snacking. Snacking interferes with the natural digestive rhythm and is not recommended. If we snack all the time, we are not giving the digestive system a chance to rest between meals. There is one exception to this: Vata Dosha is the one Dosha that might benefit from a small snack, such as fresh fruit or nuts, for energy during the mid-afternoon about 4pm, when Vata peaks and becomes aggravated.

The food and advertising industries encourage us to snack and graze all day long; if we eat properly, we really shouldn't need to snack, as we won't be hungry. However, the reality is that many of us snack even when we are not hungry; this may be to appease some emotional need, but it does not support good health.

Eat lighter foods before heavy foods. Generally, food is digested in the order in which we eat it, so it is advisable to eat light foods such as fruit before heavy foods such as red meat, which takes longer to digest. This helps to prevent food sitting in the digestive tract where it can stagnate, putrefy and cause Ama. It makes sense to eat more of the foods that are neither too light nor too heavy, including cooked vegetables and grains that go well together. Listen to your body and eat food that you can easily digest. We want to get up from the dining table feeling satisfied and energised, not heavy and stuffed as we may feel after a traditional festive meal.

Raw food and salads are difficult to digest and require more energy. We can think of the digestive system like a cooking pot: raw food takes much more energy to digest than cooked food does, where the food has already been transformed by the cooking process that makes it easier to digest.

Think about how long it takes to cook celery. A small side-salad with a dressing, oily for Vata and creamy for Pitta, is fine. But most of us benefit from restricting cold raw food to the hot summer months and eating it at lunchtime. Raw foods that have the same Gunas as Vata, being cold, dry and light, will especially aggravate Vata. Many modern diets advocate a diet high in raw foods but most of us fare better with cooked foods that are kinder to the digestive system.

Do not eat late at night. There should be a few hours between dinner and going to bed. As soon as we lie down the digestive process significantly slows, almost coming to a halt. Ensure that you do not go to bed on a full stomach. Eating a lighter early-evening dinner and reducing the use of heavy foods is kinder to our digestive system and our waistlines.

Moderate the use of stimulants, including coffee and alcohol. Instead, use water and herbal teas, especially those that are good for digestion, such as ginger. Stimulants increase Vata and aggravate the nervous system, are Rajasic in nature and disturb the mind. Alcohol is also sour and heating, which makes it very Pitta-aggravating.

Avoid ice-cold food and drink and fizzy drinks, as they shock and suppress digestion by affecting the Agni (digestive fire). This results in the digestive fire being extinguished and the system shutting down. Fizzy drinks often contain a high sugar content or artificial sweeteners that our digestion struggles with; artificial gas disturbs all Doshas and has no Prana. Natural bubbles, as in champagne, are said to be okay for Pitta and Kapha but are not recommended for Vata. Therefore, it is best to avoid these foods.

Cook with herbs and spices, which add flavour and support good digestion as well as having plenty of medicinal benefits. There are many classic herbs that reflect cooking styles from around the world, such as cinnamon and coriander from the Middle East and cumin and ginger from India. Classic food-herb pairings that complement and enhance the taste of the food include tomato with basil leaves and peas with mint. Adding herbs and spices in cooking is an easy way of enhancing digestion. Cooking with herbs and spices can also be used as an antidote to reduce possible effects of gas or bloating from vegetables in the cabbage family and legumes, making these easier to digest for Vata Dosha.

Classic Ayurveda herbs and spices to balance the Doshas:

- Vata includes cardamom, fennel and cumin seeds.
- Pitta digestive spices are the cooling and neutral spices, including cumin seeds, fennel seeds, cinnamon and coriander.

• Kapha benefit from stronger heating spices, including black pepper, ginger, fenugreek seeds, pippali (long pepper) and cumin seeds.

Starting the day with a glass of filtered water

Starting the morning with the simple routine of drinking a glass of filtered water before doing anything else has an amazing therapeutic effect in preparing the body for the day. It pacifies Vata, helps to clear toxins from the body, and alleviates constipation. Pure water is one of the best fluids that we can drink, and it is important to drink enough during the day to stay hydrated:

• Vata – 750ml of warm water. Nothing beats fresh water, so enjoy it pure.
• Pitta – 500ml of cool water. Do not be tempted to add a slice of lemon, which is sour and heating and increases Pitta. However, you could add a sprig of fresh cooling mint from the garden.
• Kapha – 300ml of hot water. You might like to add a thin slice of fresh ginger root to your morning water to liven it up a bit.

Eating mindfully

Eating mindfully is about being fully present and giving our full attention to the experience of eating and to the food itself, without being distracted by the television, mobile phone or work. It helps digestion if we are in a calm frame of mind and sit upright at a table when we eat.

There is a phrase in Ayurveda, '*Prajnaparadha*', meaning 'crimes against wisdom', where we know deep down that what we are doing is not good for us, but we obstinately do it anyway. Comfort eating is one example of this. If only we could stop for a minute and ask ourselves, 'What do I really need now?'

Food can be used to ground ourselves, especially to pacify Vata. Through the stresses of our modern world, we can easily become ungrounded, stressed and distracted; this is one of the reasons why we graze and snack. We need to find more helpful ways to ground ourselves, such as meditation, moderate exercise, Pranayama breathing and walking in nature.

Giving gratitude is also of great value, often called 'Grace' before meals – giving gratitude for our food and our shared world.

9. Dietary Advice for Dosha Prakriti

When we are well and our Doshas are in balance, this is called Prakriti. Gathering together the information we have already seen, we can now put a Dosha Prakriti diet plan together. A Prakriti diet is our diet for life: how we should eat to keep our bodies and Doshas in balance.

Your food is made up of Rasa (tastes) and the Gunas (qualities). Some of these will decrease and balance your Dosha while others will increase and aggravate your Dosha. If we eat more of the foods that suit us, we will remain balanced and healthy. You may wish to revisit Part 2 to familiarise yourself with those foods, having their different Rasas and Gunas, that are best for you.

We have also looked at how the Doshas relate to time – the seasons and the time of day. So, it's not just what we eat that matters but equally important is how we eat for our Dosha. It is important to adjust our diet for each season, enjoying eating what the season brings from what is grown locally.

Ayurveda recommends eating seasonally and we adjust our Prakriti diet with the seasons, so we eat a Vata diet in autumn and early winter, a Kapha diet in late winter and spring, and a Pitta diet in late spring and summer. This is detailed in the section on Seasonal Foods.

Eating well is obviously only one aspect of achieving good health; it is also important to look at your lifestyle as well. Stress, lack of sleep and living a life that you know doesn't suit you – whether it's where you live, relationship issues or a toxic work environment – all impact on your health. We all benefit from living with integrity and being true to ourselves. Ayurveda offers guidance on living our lives well, including daily and seasonal routines.

Diet for Vata Dosha

Vata Dosha:	
Elements	Ether (space) and air (wind)
Function	Movement
Gunas (qualities)	Dry, light, cold, rough and mobile
Season	Autumn & early winter
Time of day	2–6 am/pm
Digestion	Variable digestion
Taste	Sweet, sour, salt

Table 9.1 Vata Dosha

Structuring a diet for Vata Dosha – Vata is all about movement and, like the wind, can be variable and changeable. Vata often has a variable digestion ranging from very quick to very slow, just as the wind can go from being very blustery to very still. So, the goal of a Vata diet is to balance and reduce this variability to make it more even, ironing out the extremes.

There are two key recommendations for Vata Prakriti:

1. Eat at regular times during the day – routine is important for Vata. Don't skip meals. A good routine might be breakfast at 8am, lunch at 12.30pm and dinner at 6.30pm, so that the meals are evenly spread out during the day. Vata is pacified by food in the stomach, so this routine helps to balance Vata.

2. Vata is cold and dry and really benefits from eating warm cooking foods, especially cooked moist foods such as porridge, soup and stews, to counteract these cold dry Gunas (qualities).

The rudiments of an Ayurveda Vata diet are:

- Servings per day: 1–2 fruit, 3+ cooked vegetables, green salad, 3 whole grains, a small handful of nuts & seeds, herbal tea. Legumes 1–2 per week.

- Optional at lunchtime: 1 small serving of fish, dairy, eggs or white meat.

- Herbal tea acts as a digestive as well as supporting hydration and is a healthier alternative to black tea or coffee.

Other principles include the following:

- If you have a predominance of Vata Dosha, it is essential to follow the principles of a Vata diet in autumn and early winter, a time when Vata is most aggravated.

- Vata is also most aggravated between 2 and 6, early morning and afternoon. Ways to alleviate this include having a small, planned snack, perhaps of fruit or nuts, in mid-afternoon (say, 4pm) and a milky drink before bedtime to alleviate insomnia. A small cup of warm milk spiced with a pinch (200mg) of fresh ginger, cinnamon, cardamom or nutmeg (100mg) is a nutritious way to soothe the nerves and when taken before bed helps to promote sound sleep. Snacking should be avoided, except for these small, planned snacks.

• Vata becomes more aggravated as we get older, along with a reduced Agni (our digestive fire), when we often benefit from smaller, lighter, warmer meals.

• Vata benefits from the sweet and sour tastes and a little salt with the earth, fire and water elements that counteract Vata's light and cool nature. This includes sweet and sour tasting fruits, cooked earthy root vegetables, grains, nuts and seeds.

• Vata benefits from reducing pungent, bitter and astringent-tasting foods that have the same elements as Vata of air and ether. This includes legumes and vegetables from the cabbage family that can be drying and difficult to digest, creating wind and bloating.

• Vata is light and often has a small appetite, so it is important to ensure that every mouthful is nourishing and enjoyable. Vata often has a sensitive gut and is more susceptible to food allergies and digestive issues. Simpler, smaller meals can help with this.

• Vata is prone to dryness and constipation, so adding more fluid and good fats and oils to the diet really helps with this. Oil, nuts, seeds, nut butters, avocado, butter and ghee are unctuous and stop the dryness. Unctuous foods are those that are slightly oily and liquid.

• Limit dry, rough foods like crispbread, dry crackers, muesli or granola breakfast cereal, dried fruit, soya and raw vegetables and salad that will exacerbate the dry, rough Gunas (qualities) of Vata.

• Vata often benefits from having a little animal protein in the diet, especially oily fish, eggs, chicken and wild game.

• Very cold drinks and foods, including ice cream and fizzy drinks, can be very aggravating for Vata.

• Stimulants such as coffee and alcohol can be very destabilizing for Vata.

• Start the day with a large glass (1 litre) of warm filtered water.

• Good culinary herbs and spices for Vata include cardamom, fennel and cumin seeds.

Vata Food Groups

Fruit

Good	Most sweet and sour fruit are good for Vata Fruits that include the astringent taste – bananas and raspberries, but ensure they are really ripe Apples are best eaten cooked, especially warm stewed apple Dried fruit is best soaked or cooked
Limit	Melons – hard to digest Cranberries – astringent

Vegetables

Good	Most vegetables have a sweet neutral taste and are good for Vata Avocado – a small portion, as heavy and hard to digest
Limit	Cabbage family: cabbage, Brussels sprouts, cauliflower and radish that are astringent and drying, or antidote with herbs and spices Solanaceae vegetables: potatoes,

	peppers, aubergine, tomatoes, chillies Raw and dry vegetables and salads – can be difficult to digest Mushrooms – astringent and dry

Grains

Good	Most moist cooked grains are fairly neutral: either slightly cooling or mildly warming served as a breakfast cereal or bread, incorporated into a soup or stew or accompanying a main meal.
Limit	Dry cereals; muesli, granola – can be antidoted with warm milk to make them more balancing for Vata Rice cakes, crisp bread – can be antidoted with moist oily spreads such as hummus and nut butter to make them more balancing for Vata. Yeasted commercial breads Processed white rice and wheat

Legumes – pulses and beans

Good	Mung beans and Aduki beans are best for Vata
Limit	All other legumes

Nuts and seeds

Good	All nuts and seeds are good for Vata in small amounts
Limit	No limit

Dairy

Good	All dairy produce is good for Vata
Limit	Ice cream – cold

Animal produce

Good	All meat and fish are nutritious for Vata, including wild game and oily fish
Limit	Red meat: beef, lamb and pork

Oils

Good	Most natural vegetable oils are beneficial for Vata
Limit	Processed oils and margarine

Sweeteners

Good	Natural sweeteners: maple syrup, raw honey, jaggery
Limit	Processed sugar: granulated and brown sugar Artificial sweeteners

Beverages

Good	Filtered water Herbal teas (sweet and spicy)
Limit	Alcohol

	Coffee, tea Iced cold or artificial soft and fizzy drinks

Herbs and spices

Good	All herbs and spices are good for Vata, especially cardamom, fennel and cumin seeds
Limit	Chillies

Diet for Pitta Dosha

Pitta Dosha:	
Elements	Fire and water
Function	Transformation and digestion
Gunas (qualities)	Slightly oily, penetrating, hot, light and spreading
Season	Late spring and summer
Time of day	10–2 am/pm
Metabolism	Strong digestion
Taste	Sweet, bitter, astringent

Table 9.2 Pitta Dosha

Structuring a diet for Pitta Dosha – Pitta is all about transformation, including digestion. People with a predominant Pitta Dosha tend to have a strong digestion due to the heating, fiery nature of Pitta and have no problem eating virtually any food; they can become angry (hangry!) when a meal is missed.

The goal of a Pitta diet is to keep Pitta's fire under control; we don't want to put the fire out but equally we don't want it getting out of control and spreading to create more problems in the body. So, we don't want to give the digestive fire any foods that will ignite the flames.

There are two key recommendations for Pitta Prakriti:

1. Eat three equally sized meals a day. It is important to eat enough at mealtimes to avoid

getting hungry between meals. Be honest with yourself and have enough food to satisfy you until the next meal. For you it is miserable being hungry. Make sure that work schedules or exercise routines do not dishonour your need to look after yourself.

2. Pitta is the principle of fire and is hot, light, sharp and oily; so, reduce the use of hot, pungent spices and sharp, acidic, sour flavours to balance Pitta. Examples of these are sour fruits such as lemons; oil and fried foods, and alcohol and foods that are fermented or contain yeast. These foods all contain the fire element and are heating. The exceptions to this are olive oil, coconut oil, ghee and butter, which are identified as cooling fats.

The rudiments of an Ayurveda Pitta diet are:

• Servings per day: 2 fruit, 4+ vegetables, side salad with a creamy dressing, 3–5 whole grains, herbal tea. Legumes 3-4 per week.

• Optional at lunchtime: 1 small serving of fish, dairy, eggs or white meat.

• Herbal tea acts as a digestive as well as supporting hydration and is a healthier alternative to black tea or coffee.

Other principles include the following:

- If you have a predominance of Pitta Dosha, it is essential to follow the principles of a Pitta diet in late spring and summer, when Pitta is most aggravated.

- Pitta is also most aggravated between 10 and 2 am and pm. Agni, the digestive fire, is at its strongest at midday. Using the principles of Ayurveda, if you wish to indulge, for example with eating some red meat (which is heavy and hard to digest) or a glass of wine (which is heating and acidic), this is best enjoyed at lunchtime when the Agni will help you to digest these better.

- Pitta is more aggravated during our adult years. It is important to remember the principles of a Pitta diet: balancing a stronger digestion with reducing the foods, especially the heating, sour and pungent tastes that aggravate Pitta, along with managing our Pitta characteristics that can lead to symptoms of hyperacidity and heart problems.

- Pitta benefits from the sweet, bitter and astringent-tasting foods that are cooling and do not include the fire element. The major part of the diet should come from the sweet taste plus a portion of both bitter and astringent tastes into the daily diet. This could be a portion of bitter greens and astringent legumes or vegetables.

• Pitta benefits from restricting the sour taste to about one portion a day, and significantly reducing the salt and pungent tastes that have the heating fire element that is already present in Pitta. This includes sour fruits, fermented foods, alcohol and hot, pungent spices.

• Pitta has a strong digestion, often benefits from larger portion sizes and has no problem eating virtually any food. However, Pitta can be sensitive to raw onions and to plants from the Solanaceae family: potatoes, aubergines, tomatoes, peppers and chillies.

• Pitta is slightly oily so it helps to limit oils and oily foods such as nuts and meat that can exacerbate this quality in Pitta.

• Pitta benefits from foods that have cooling and drying Gunas (qualities) to counteract Pitta's heating, oily nature. This includes cooling fruits, vegetables, herbs, mushrooms, astringent legumes and breakfast granola.

• Pitta, when aggravated, can be prone to hyperacidity and acid reflux. Pungent, heating spices and stimulants such as alcohol, coffee and fruit juice can exacerbate this. Eating a more neutral diet avoiding extreme tastes and overly light or heavy foods helps to support digestion.

• Start the day with half a litre of cool filtered water.

- Try to avoid snacking.

- Good culinary herbs and spices for Pitta include the cooling and neutral spices: cumin seeds, fennel seeds and coriander.

Pitta Food Groups

Fruit

Good	Sweet fruits are best for Pitta
Limit	Sour fruits: lemon, lime and grapefruit

Vegetables

Good	Most vegetables have a sweet neutral taste and are good for Pitta
Limit	Heating pungent vegetables: raw onion, radish Avocado – oily, warm and heavy Solanaceae vegetables: potatoes, peppers, aubergine, tomatoes, chillies

Grains

Good	Most grains are fairly neutral; either slightly cooling or mildly warming
Limit	Processed white rice and wheat Yeasted bread

Legumes – pulses and beans

Good	All beans are good in moderation
Limit	Peanuts (which are a legume, rather than a nut) are oily

Nuts and seeds

Good	Coconut is sweet and cooling
Limit	All other nuts and seeds – oily

Dairy

Good	Cooling dairy produce is good for Pitta
Limit	Fermented, sour warm dairy: hard cheese, goat's cheese, kefir, yoghurt and sour cream Ice cream – cold

Animal produce

Good	Most meat and freshwater fish is nutritious for Pitta
Limit	Red meat: beef, lamb and pork Duck Salt-water fish and shellfish

Oils

Good	Olive oil and coconut oil are cooling and best for Pitta Small quantities of most natural vegetable oils are fine, although they are warming
Limit	Processed oils and margarine Fried foods

Sweeteners

Good	Natural sweeteners: maple syrup, jaggery, raw honey
Limit	Processed sugar: granulated and brown sugar Artificial sweeteners

Beverages

Good	Filtered water Herbal teas (sweet)
Limit	Alcohol Sour fruit juices or teas Pungent spicy herbal teas Iced cold or artificial soft and fizzy drinks

Herbs and spices

Good	Cool herbs and spices are good for Pitta, especially coriander and mint Mild spices: fennel, cardamom, cumin and turmeric – fresh is best when it is available
Limit	Hot pungent spices including black pepper, cayenne, chillies, horseradish, mustard and raw garlic

Diet for Kapha Dosha

Kapha Dosha:	
Elements	Earth and water
Function	Cohesion and stability
Gunas (qualities)	Oily, cool, heavy, slow
Season	Late winter & early spring
Time of day	6–10 am/pm
Digestion	Slow and steady
Taste	Pungent, bitter and astringent

Table 9.3 Kapha Dosha

Structuring a diet for Kapha Dosha – Kapha is all about cohesion and stability in the body. Kapha's digestion is influenced by the heavy earth and water elements that create a slow and steady digestion. Kapha need the least amount of food and are often not hungry, although they love their food. The goal of a Kapha diet is to enliven the digestive system.

There are two key recommendations for Kapha Prakriti:

1. Kapha time is from 6 to 10 in the morning and evening, which is when they want lighter meals, especially at breakfast. We have the saying, 'Eat breakfast like a King'; however, that's not the case for Kapha, who often benefit from not eating first thing in the morning. They often get hungry later in the morning at about 10.30 to 11.00 am, after Kapha time, which is when they are advised to eat breakfast. They often do well on seasonal fruit or

just a digestive tea, unless they are hungry or are having a very physically active day. If they eat earlier when they are not hungry, Ama is formed. Most Kapha types are more energised by eating breakfast later or not at all.

2. Kapha fare better when they eat less and choose lighter foods, and where possible make lunch the main meal of the day and the evening meal a smaller, lighter meal. A good question for a Kapha person to ask themselves is, 'Am I hungry?' – it might be that you are thirsty or just need a break to give yourself a rest from what you are doing.

The rudiments of a Kapha diet are:

• Servings per day: 1 fruit, 3+ vegetables, side salad, 2 whole grains, herbal tea. Legumes 3-4 per week.

• Optional at lunchtime: 1 small serving of fish, eggs or white meat - 4 per week.

• Herbal tea acts as a digestive as well as supporting hydration and is a healthier alternative to black tea or coffee.

Other principles include the following:

• If you have a predominance of Kapha Dosha it is essential to follow the principles of a Kapha diet in the later winter and spring when Kapha is most aggravated.

- Kapha is also most aggravated between 6 and 10 both in the morning and evening so, as well as following the breakfast advice above, it often helps to have a smaller, lighter evening meal. The main meal should be at lunchtime, which is away from Kapha time. It is also the time where our digestive fire is highest, and this will really help with digestion.

- Kapha benefits from eating more pungent and bitter tasting foods that do not contain the earth or water elements, as well as some astringent taste that does not contain the water element. These foods include heating pungent spices and a portion of bitter leafy greens and astringent vegetables or legumes daily. All these tastes contain the air element, which is drying; additionally, pungent is heating, which counteracts the coolness of Kapha.

- Kapha benefits from eating a little less of the sweet and sour tastes. However, these tastes still make up about 80% of the diet, which has much less of the salt taste.

- Kapha is heavy, so benefits from eating neutral and lighter foods to counteract this heaviness. This includes eating less heavy animal and dairy produce and eating more lighter, green leafy vegetables. Kapha really benefits from eating a more plant-based diet with lots of different vegetables. Limit the amount of fresh fruit in the diet, as this is sweet and liquid.

- Likewise, Kapha is oily and cool, so benefits from limiting oils, nuts, seeds and oily foods in the diet and eating more drying, lighter and hotter foods.

- Kapha can be prone to weight gain and needs to be mindful of how much they eat, so reduce foods, including sugar, wheat and fats, that can pile on the calories and increase blood sugar levels. Eating more pungent and heating digestive herbs and spices can also help to stimulate and aid digestion.

- Dairy products are generally best avoided as they are cold and heavy, create mucus and increase Kapha Dosha.

- Kapha really benefits from not snacking, as this interferes with the natural digestive rhythm.

- When Kapha is aggravated, digestion slows down and produces excess mucus that suppresses the digestive fire. At these times it is even more important to avoid snacking, eat breakfast later, exercise more, eat less and avoid dairy, yoghurt, ice cream and cold foods.

- Kapha love their food but need the least amount of food and often don't recognise when they are full. Eating mindfully and listening for the first 'burp' can help with this. Kapha often do well on two meals a day.

- Start the day with a mug of hot filtered water.

- Good culinary herbs for Kapha are the more heating, pungent spices including black pepper, dry ginger, Pippali long pepper, cumin seeds, cardamom, cinnamon and fennel.

Kapha Food Groups

Fruit

Good	A small portion of fruit daily. Apples, cranberries (astringent) and dried fruit are best
Limit	Heavy sweet fruits; bananas, dates

Vegetables

Good	Most vegetables are good for Kapha, especially those from the cabbage family (astringent)
Limit	Avocado, cucumber and sweet potato

Grains

Good	Most grains are fairly neutral; either slightly cooling or mildly warming, especially rye and barley
Limit	Processed white rice and wheat Yeasted bread

Legumes – pulses and beans

Good	All beans are good in moderation
Limit	Peanuts

Nuts and seeds

Good	Seeds are better than nuts for Kapha but keep the portion size very small
Limit	All nuts increase Kapha

Dairy

Good	Small amount of soya milk is a good alternative for Kapha, who often find dairy foods mucus forming Ghee is good for cooking, to replace oil
Limit	Limit dairy produce including milk, cream, cheese and ice cream

Animal produce

Good	Most white meat, fish and eggs
Limit	Red meat: beef, lamb and pork

Oils

Good	Very small quantities of most natural vegetable oils
Limit	Processed oils and margarine Fried foods

Sweeteners

Good	Very small amounts of natural sweeteners; raw honey is best Cinnamon spice makes a nice alternative to sweeteners, especially with stewed apple
Limit	Maple syrup (cooling) Processed sugar: granulated and brown sugar Artificial sweeteners

Beverages

Good	Filtered water Herbal teas (spicy) – ginger
Limit	Alcohol Milk Iced cold or artificial soft and fizzy drinks

Herbs and spices

Good	All herbs and spices are good for Kapha, especially pungent heating spices: black pepper, ginger, horseradish, cardamom, cumin, turmeric
Limit	Salt

Note – The rudiments of a Prakriti diet are guidelines only and not prescriptive. Other Ayurveda practitioners' views may differ, and you need to vary any diet to suit you as an individual.

10. What to Eat

In looking at diets for each Dosha, we have addressed how to put the components of a diet together but have not specified what dishes to eat. Many Ayurveda cookbooks have a strong emphasis on Indian-style cookery, as this is where Ayurveda originates from. However lovely this food might be, this is not to say that this style of eating will necessarily suit us long term, unless this is our heritage.

It is more important to understand how to use the principles of Ayurveda to identify when to eat, how much to eat, and which Rasa (tastes) and Gunas (qualities) suit you best, rather than feeling that you are required to eat an Asian-style diet.

Evidence shows us that the typical British diet is not proving to be good for our health. Whether it's eating too many ready meals, too much British stodge or trying to emulate television cookery programmes, it's not working.

So, one option is to look to the Mediterranean diet, which is always being promoted as a healthy one, especially for cardiovascular health.

The rudiments of a Mediterranean diet are:

- Servings per day: 1-2 fruit, 4+ vegetables, 4-6 whole grains, 1-2 dairy including cheese and yoghurt, a handful of nuts and seeds. Cook with herbs and spices, use olive oil as the principal source of fat.
- Servings per week: 2+ fish, 2 white poultry, 2-4 eggs, 2+ legumes, 2 potatoes.
- Less than once a week: red meat, dessert and sweets – have small amounts and for special occasions.
- Drink water and herbal infusions.

(Adapted from Bach-Fraig et al. (2011) Mediterranean diet pyramid today, Science and cultural updates. Public Health Nutrition. *14 (12a) 2274–84)*

The rudiments of the Mediterranean diet have much in common with the Ayurveda diet, with a greater emphasis on good-quality fresh plant-based foods and less red meat and sweets. Especially for people who come from a starting point of a very conventionally British diet, the Mediterranean diet provides an easy way to construct a healthier diet and is closer to our own heritage. With an understanding of Ayurveda, we can easily adapt the Mediterranean diet for our Dosha, taking account of portion sizes, Rasas (tastes), Gunas (qualities) and the seasons. This avoids it becoming a one-size-fits-all diet, which is not what Ayurveda is about.

Changing your eating habits is a personal journey, making choices and changes that work for you. As the Rishis of ancient times knew, it makes sense to be more in touch with the natural world around us, be more curious of where our food comes from and how it is sourced, and then observe how you feel after you have eaten a meal. Do you feel energised or heavy? What works for you? The skill is often in finding the single small change that makes all the difference and that then motivates you to make some more changes.

Seasonal food

We are designed to eat foods from our natural local environment, which includes eating foods that match the seasons. Nature corresponds with the Doshas, and there are good reasons why cool, sweet berries are summer fruits, while root vegetables are at their best in the autumn and early winter when our bodies are getting ready for the cold of winter.

As we have already identified, the Doshas relate to the seasons, and we are encouraged to change our diet with the time of year. By doing this we are balancing the Dosha that is strongest in time. However, this still needs to be nuanced for our predominant Dosha Prakriti. If your Dosha Prakriti is shared by two Doshas, it is advisable to adjust your diet accordingly. Details of how to do this have been given in chapter 2: *Seasonal diet for mixed Dosha types*.

Kapha is the season of spring, when the earth is waking up after the hibernation of winter. We hopefully feel more energised and are ready to eat a slightly lighter diet and embrace more of the bitter, astringent and pungent tastes. It can also be a time of spring allergies, which can be reduced by a Kapha-reducing diet, including less dairy produce, heavy foods and oils and fatty foods. It's a time when we're ready to enjoy the new season's produce of rhubarb and asparagus.

Pitta is the season of summer, when the days are lengthening, the weather is hot, and we are ready to eat lighter, cooler foods. This is the season of summer berries and salads, with less meat, oils, pungent spices and heating sour-tasting foods.

Vata is the season of autumn, when we're ready to change our diet to enjoy more warming, heavy, unctuous foods again with vegetable soups and stews as the days shorten and the weather gets colder. We are no longer interested in eating dry, light and cold foods but want something that will give keep us grounded and warm us as we head towards winter. It is a time to enjoy the abundance of the harvest with more grains and earthy root vegetables.

For many of us this is a logical and natural way to eat, especially if we enjoy home cooking, grow our own vegetables or shop at a farmers market that promotes what is fresh and in season. However, supermarkets and food manufacturers encourage us to ignore this wisdom and tempt us to eat whatever we like whenever we like, which is not how we are designed to eat for our health.

All these Dosha diets encourage moderation and eating in harmony with our local environment. Ayurveda encourages us to change what we eat with the seasons; so, for example, even if you have a Pitta or a Kapha Dosha Prakriti you may want to change to a Vata-style diet as we move into autumn, with less cooling and more warming meals.

However, it is important to listen to your own body and make adjustments that are right for your Prakriti Dosha throughout the year. For example, if you have a predominantly Pitta Dosha, it may well be that you still want to eat slightly larger meals to ensure that you don't get hungry before the next meal, and you should only slightly increase the amount of sour-tasting foods you eat in Vata season, otherwise you risk increasing your Pitta Dosha and creating Vikriti. If you have a Kapha Dosha you may still benefit from eating breakfast later, after Kapha time.

Refer to Appendix 2 for a guide to seasonal British fruit and vegetables.

80:20 Rule

When we are well and our Doshas are balanced, we can afford to deviate from the Dosha diet occasionally without much adverse effect. Ayurveda is realistic and allows for some flexibility; whether it's for a celebration or times when it is more difficult to make the right choices, as for instance when we are away from home or for an ingredient we absolutely love. Relaxing the rules for up to five meals a week or twenty percent of the time whilst aiming for an Ayurveda diet can still support positive results and is part of the Ayurveda philosophy of balance and moderation without being too rigid and obsessive about your diet. A stricter regime is required when we are not well or are imbalanced (Vikriti).

11. Dietary Advice for Dosha Vikriti

Vikriti

Vikriti is when one or more of the Doshas are out of balance and are covering up the original Prakriti. Vikriti is a term used to describe any imbalance, whether it be stress, indigestion, insomnia, a mild cold or a major chronic disease.

A trained Ayurveda practitioner can diagnose which Dosha is causing the imbalance or illness. Additionally, an imbalance when left untreated can spread to create imbalance and disease to all three Doshas.

As a general guide it is usually your strongest Dosha that goes out of balance first. However, our modern way of living creates a predominance of Vata aggravation.

In this book I have focused on an introduction to Ahara Chikitsa – Food as Medicine – and I have not gone into the details of Ayurveda anatomy and physiology, pathology, diagnosis or treatment of disease.

Ayurveda practitioners do not diagnose Dosha Vikriti in isolation. Before prescribing an individual therapeutic treatment, they also consider whether there is Ama (toxins) in the body, how balanced the Agni (digestive fire) is and your strength (*Bala*) – whether a person has a strong constitution or is showing signs of weakness or fragility.

It is also advisable to use a Vikriti diet for convalescence, to aid recovery from an illness, after major surgery or after a traditional Ayurveda Pancha Karma therapy to reignite Agni. A convalescent diet has very much gone out of favour in today's world, but eating very simple light and nourishing foods are so valuable to reignite the Agni (digestive fire) and restore health.

Convalescence means to regain health and relates to the period of time to make a complete recovery. As we have seen in Long Covid, an initial recovery from the infection needs to be followed by a time of healing, for the body to recover after the crisis. Within that there may be a need for rehabilitation, of relearning how to 'get back on the road again', including learning how to pace yourself and manage energy well. People with mental health crises also often benefit from a place and space to heal, a place of rest and safety. In this process we need kindness and compassion from ourselves and others.

Recognise your food enemies. For many people, these might be grains (especially wheat), dairy (particularly A1 milk from Ayrshire, Friesian, Holstein and British Shorthorn cattle), sugar, coffee, and vegetables from the Solanaceae family. Taking a rest from these foods allows your body to restore its balance and health.

Some Vikriti illnesses benefit from adding and/or eliminating certain foods. For example, people experiencing irritable bowel syndrome may be advised by their doctor to use a low FODMAP diet (meaning foods that are low in carbohydrates that are Fermentable, Oligosaccharides, Disaccharides, Monosaccharides and Polyols); or someone with type two diabetes may be recommended to choose foods with a low glycaemic index to reduce the impact on blood sugar levels. This is a specialism of using food medicinally that is best undertaken with a health practitioner and is not covered in this book.

I would also stress the importance of removing Ama from the body, as according to Ayurveda all disease begins with Ama. This is the first, early stage of the disease process, which we often don't recognise or ignore for years and which if left unchecked can go on to create chronic degenerative diseases. In ancient times you paid the Ayurveda doctor to keep you well, not leaving it until you were ill before visiting them.

Vikriti diet

A Vikriti diet is a diet aimed at bringing the Doshas back into balance.

If you are having a day or a few days when you are feeling off colour, it is advisable to eat a diet for your Dosha Prakriti. So, if you have a Kapha Prakriti, even if we are in the summer Pitta season you should follow your Kapha Dosha diet, with no variations except those listed in the following pages. It is usually our predominant Dosha that goes out of balance first, so this is the Dosha we treat first.

However, if you are feeling stressed or anxious and it is obvious that it is Vata Dosha that is imbalanced and out of sorts, then follow a Vata diet, again with no variations except those listed in the following pages.

It is advised to follow a Vikriti diet until the Dosha has been brought back into balance, which may be just for a few days but could be for much longer.

If your health issues have gone beyond mild imbalances and they are now showing as serious illness including autoimmune or degenerative disorders, it is likely that the disease has spread into all three Doshas and is now more complicated to treat. This is when you are advised to speak to a doctor or Ayurveda practitioner, who can prescribe a more personalised treatment plan for you.

When we are unwell or recovering from an operation, we need to eat to reignite our Agni, our digestive fire, and remove the cause of the Dosha imbalance.

Pancha Karma is a specialist Ayurveda therapy treatment carried out in a clinical environment to cleanse the body and balance the Doshas. These strong purification treatments shut down the digestion. It is essential to spend time (usually seven days) reigniting the Agni (digestive fire) after a Pancha Karma treatment.

Suggestions for a Vikriti diet:

Firstly, it is important to eat a wholefood diet, avoid processed foods and apply the other recommendations outlined in this book to promote health.

Follow the advice without deviation for the Dosha that is showing signs of being most imbalanced. For example, for a Pitta Vikriti diet you should follow the guidelines for a Pitta diet outlined above and limit foods that taste sour and pungent, as they are hot and can exacerbate Pitta Dosha, which is already hot and out of balance.

- Only eat when hungry.
- Eat smaller meals.
- Eat lighter foods.
- Avoid cold raw foods, which are difficult to digest.

- Eat meals with fewer ingredients.
- Keep the diet fairly neutral in taste.
- Drink digestive tea.

Menu suggestions

We follow the guidelines in the Prakriti Dosha diets above for the Dosha that is most out of balance. It is advisable to choose lighter, blander meals such as porridge for breakfast with seasonal fruit, and Kitchari or soup with non-yeasted bread for lunch and dinner.

Ideally, it makes sense to be flexible, to adapt your diet and your day to consider how you feel. It is not heroic to just ignore a headache, stress or the effect of a bad night's sleep without being able to be kind to yourself and to make a few adjustments to support your wellbeing. Sometimes small adjustments to our diet and lifestyle can correct an imbalance before it becomes a serious issue.

12. How to Improve Digestion

Causes of imbalanced Agni

The major cause of imbalanced Agni, our digestive fire, is an aggravation of the Doshas. As we looked at in Chapter 3 Agni – digestive fire, Agni is managed by the Doshas, and therefore balancing and correcting Dosha function is how we manage digestion in the body.

For instance, a Vata person eating a Vata-aggravating diet – such as having too many cold, light salads, drinking fizzy diet drinks and snacking on dry crisps all day – creates digestive problems. This commonly show up as wind and bloating or constipation.

There are many potential causes of the Agni becoming imbalanced, including:

Any of the causes above can have an adverse effect on the Doshas and this in turn affects the Agni, our digestive fire. When we do have an imbalance in our Dosha and Agni, it is important to look for the cause.

This is where a personalised diet plan is so important to balance your Dosha and Agni.

Practical ways to improve Agni

Here are a few simple but effective suggestions to increase our Agni.

- Before meals, eat a thin slice of raw ginger root, sprinkled with lime juice and rock salt.
- Avoid drinking excessive amounts of water, especially during and after meals. Just sipping a little water whilst eating is sufficient.
- Avoid cold or iced drinks.
- Only eat when you feel hungry, and don't over-eat.
- Chew food well.
- Chew a few roasted fennel seeds after a meal.
- Avoid excessive consumption of coffee.
- Ayurveda recommends walking as a gentle exercise to improve circulation and enhance Agni.
- Cook with culinary digestive spices.

Agni diet

This is a classic Ayurveda protocol used in Pancha Karma therapies that we can adapt (as shown below) to reignite the Agni after major surgery, when our digestive fire will have been shocked and temporarily shut down.

Stage 1 Rice water:

1 cup of basmati rice cooked well
with 14 cups of water
Meal one – just drink the rice water.

Stage 2 Rice soup:

1 cup of basmati rice with 4 cups of water, a little natural sugar, ghee and a few light spices such as black pepper, ginger, turmeric, cumin and fennel. Cook until the rice is soft.
Use for one day.

Stage 3 Mung bean and rice soup:

¾ cup of basmati rice, ¼ cup of mung beans, 4 cups of water and a little ginger
Use for next two days.
Final stage Kitchari

How long it takes to return the Agni to normal will depend on the strength of the person who is recovering. It will normally return to normal within three or four days.

If you are in hospital for major surgery or with a serious illness, it may be advisable to order the soup and Kitchari dish (which should be available on the Asian menu) for the first few meals to support your Agni if you are unable to control your own diet.

Once the appetite is restored, we can start to introduce simple Sattvic dishes such as porridge, simple soup, rice with sautéed vegetables and a few spices for the next few days of convalescence.

Digestive herbs

Using digestive herbs and spices with meals will help to improve, correct and balance digestion. Digestive spices have *plant* Agni that supports *our* Agni. We need to ensure that the herbs we use have the correct Gunas (qualities) to support both our Dosha and our digestion. Vata benefit from warming spices, Pitta benefit from cooling or slightly warming herbs and Kapha benefit from more heating spices.

Dipana herbs are those that improve and balance our digestion. They are normally taken with a meal as a quarter-teaspoon of lightly ground medicinal-grade powdered herbs with a little warm water. Sometimes it is appropriate to use just a single herb but more commonly we use a traditional formula for each Dosha. Some of the most common Dipana herbs are cardamom (Vata), fennel (Vata and Pitta), cumin (Vata, Pitta and Kapha), coriander (Pitta), ginger (Kapha), black pepper (Kapha) and fenugreek (Kapha). We use equal amounts of each herb in the formula. Traditionally this is taken before main meals for all Dosha types. However, using herbs and spices in cooking and drinking herbal teas also work well.

Pachana herbs are those that are used to support digestion and to remove Ama. They are normally a balanced formula, individually made by an

Ayurveda herbalist, that includes primary, stronger herbs to literally scrape and burn the Ama from the walls of the digestive tract along with gentler, secondary herbs to balance and support the primary herbs and digestion. A blend of about ten different herbs is personalised to support each individual, and the spice blend used for each Dosha is different.

Ways to remove Ama (toxins)

Firstly, we need to classify the type of Ama by examination of the tongue and from a Dosha questionnaire; then we treat accordingly for that particular Dosha with the right:

- herbs
- diet
- digestive tea
- exercise.

Anti-Ama cleansing diet

This short-term cleansing diet is designed to help remove Ama from the body. Use an anti-Ama diet:

- when where there are clear signs of Ama
- as a preventative measure either annually or seasonally
- as part of a fasting programme.

This diet should not be followed if you are frail, underweight, unwell or ungrounded. Nor should it be used by pregnant women or children without medical supervision. If you experience side-effects of feeling unwell, lack of energy or restlessness, stop this diet and seek gentler alternative therapies.

How to use the anti-Ama diet:

- It is usually safe to use for 3 days or as guided by an Ayurveda practitioner.
- If you are working and find it difficult to follow this diet full-time, you could follow the anti-Ama diet for breakfast and supper and eat what is available normally for your Prakriti at lunchtime.

What is an anti-Ama diet?

This simple detoxification diet is based on fresh whole foods with culinary herbs and spices to support digestion. Modify your choice of foods according to your Dosha, appetite and lifestyle.

- Fruit: eat a small amount.
- Vegetables: eat seasonal, organic, cooked vegetables but choose only one or two for each meal, e.g. one root vegetable and one green vegetable. Cruciferous vegetables (broccoli, Brussels sprouts, cauliflower, kale and cabbage) are especially good as they support healthy liver function and detoxification. Avoid using vegetables from the Solanaceae family. Steamed vegetables are good. Home-made soup is a good option.
- Grains: include whole gluten-free grains. Kitchari

is a good choice when made with basmati rice or quinoa.

• Beans: only use Kitchari made with mung dhal or adzuki beans.

• Ghee in small quantities, or sesame oil or olive oil for vegans.

• Raw honey in small amounts – ½ teaspoon a day.

• Culinary spices: all spices are good.

• Drinks: mild herbal digestive teas.

How to avoid or reduce Ama

• Make meals simpler and lighter.

• Eat real unprocessed food, free from pesticides and other chemicals.

• Eat smaller meals with plenty of fresh fruit, vegetables and wholegrains.

• Do not overeat.

• Make sure there is a three-hour gap between your last meal and going to bed.

• Eat regularly.

• Eat slowly and chew well – eat mindfully.

• Leave 4-6 hours between meals and don't eat until the previous meal has been digested.

• Do not eat if you are not hungry.

• If you are stressed and adrenaline is flowing, you will not be hungry; avoid food short-term and take some digestive herbs.

• Do one thing at a time – only eat; do not read, watch TV, etc.

- It is important to make a point of tasting your food.
- No cold liquids, ice or raw foods, except a light side salad.
- Practise Pranayama breathing.
- Take adequate exercise – walking, yoga.
- Sit down when you eat; relax, stay calm and do not talk a lot.
- It is also important to have good dental hygiene and to brush your teeth regularly to prevent the build-up of bacteria in the mouth.

Digestive tea

Digestive tea is excellent for balancing digestion, cleansing the body and removing Ama. Every Ayurveda practitioner will have their own digestive tea formula passed down from their teacher. This is a blend of gentle culinary herbs, often infused with fresh ginger root. The formula will be blended for your individual Dosha and digestive needs, or a practitioner can give you the formula for you to make it yourself. It is a gentle but effective way of improving digestion and removing Ama from the digestive tract.

Digestive tea blending is an art form in its own right. It is worth taking the time to work with an Ayurveda practitioner to understand which herbs are right for you depending on your Dosha balance, age and state of health. For those who are more creative there are books on how to make fresh digestive teas to inspire you, including *Cleanse Nurture Restore with Herbal Tea* by Sebastian Pole, and these teas will have more Prana and vitality than processed herbal and fruit teas bought from the supermarket.

We would all benefit from having more digestive teas in our diet. It is a wonderful way to hydrate ourselves and support our digestion.

Ginger Tea Recipe

Vaidya Atreya Smith has kindly given me permission to include this excellent recipe for ginger tea.

The blend of herbs in this formula is designed to increase the function of digestion, cleanse the body, and remove Ama (toxins).

It can safely be used any time that your digestion needs balancing or as a formula to remove Ama from the body. This is also beneficial whenever your digestion has been compromised, whether by medical procedures, antibiotics or ill health. This formula can safely be used for up to a year to remove Ama from the body.

<u>Spices for Ginger Tea</u>

Vata	Pitta	Kapha	Spices*
1	1	1	Cumin (Cumimum cyminum)
1	1	1	Cardamon (Elettaria cardamomum)
0	1	0	Coriander (Coriandrum sativum)
1	0	1	Fenugreek (Trigonella foenum-graecum) *Avoid in pregnancy
0	1	1	Cinnamon (Cinnamomum zeylanicum)
1	1	1	Fennel (Foeniculum vuglare)
0	0	1	Ginger (Zingiber officinale)

Table 12.1 Digestive tea formula

*Organic medicinal grade powdered Spices (1 = 1 part – use equal parts by weight 0 = do not include in formula)

I recommend making this up as a blend following the correct formula and put it in a dry clean glass jar with a lid and store it in a dark, dry place.

Instructions

- Take ¼ to ½ inch (7-14mm) of peeled and chopped fresh root ginger and bring it to the boil in a saucepan with 1 litre of filtered drinking water
- Simmer the ginger so that it just very gently bubbles on the surface of the water for 10 to 20 minutes
- Turn off the heat
- Add 2-3 grams of the powered spice mix, as detailed above (about 2 level teaspoons)
- Cover the saucepan with a lid and leave for 20 minutes for the spices to infuse
- Transfer it into a thermos flask, so that you can sip it throughout the day. It is recommended to drink about 100ml at a time during the day.

Simplified instructions

If this feels too onerous you can simply add the ½" fresh peeled and chopped ginger root and 2-3 grams powdered spice mix to 1 litre of boiling water in a thermos flask and leave to infuse during the day. This obviously isn't the intended method but is a good compromise when you are short of time and energy.

13. How to Eat From an Ayurveda Perspective

Ayurvedic food combining

When too many foods with different tastes, energies and Gunas are combined, our digestive fire can sometimes become overloaded. This is especially the case in Dosha Vikriti when we are out of balance or in a diseased state, as our Agni will already be compromised.

These same foods, when eaten separately, might however stimulate Agni and be more easily digested.

Where there is Ama (toxins) and poor digestion, you are encouraged to have simpler meals with fewer different foods together in a meal. However, you are still encouraged to eat a wide variety of plant-based foods in your diet over the course of a week, but not all together in the same meal. The exception to this is when different food ingredients are cooked together as in a soup or stew, where the cooking process creates a more balanced homogenous dish that is easier to digest.

- Vata types tolerate the fewest number of food combinations.

• Pitta types do better with moderately rich food and light spicing.
• Kapha types require light food with stronger hot spices.

Classic Ayurveda list

This is a classic Ayurveda list of foods that do not mix well together. This draws together a number of different factors: the Gunas, qualities of food, tastes and particularly the lightness and heaviness of foods.

Food or food group	**Does not mix with:**
Ice-cold liquids	Anything
Complex carbohydrates	Eggs, dairy, fruits Can mix cooked grains with milk
Eggs	Cheese, fish, fruit, milk, red meat
Fruit	Anything
Honey	Ghee
Lemons	Cucumber, milk, tomato, yoghurt
Melons	Anything
Milk	Eggs, fish, red meat, sour foods, yeast breads
Solanaceae vegetables (potato, tomato, aubergine, pepper, chillies)	Cucumber, melon, milk, yoghurt
Yoghurt	Cheese, fish, mango, milk, melon, meat and sour fruits

Table 13.1 Ayurveda food combining list

Antidoting (counteracting Gunas)

Antidoting is where a substance with Gunas (qualities) that are opposite to those of a particular food is added to it to balance, help counteract and alleviate some of its negative effects on a Dosha. Antidoting is a really useful tool and means that you do not have to give up something you love – you just change its Gunas or attributes. Often we do this naturally, but Ayurveda gives us a fresh perspective on why this is not just useful for flavour and texture. Here are some examples.

- Most fruit or fruit juices can be balanced or antidoted with warm, sweet spices such as ginger, cloves, cardamom, cinnamon and nutmeg. Cooking fruit also helps.
- Green leafy salad leaves that are cold, dry and bitter will aggravate Vata, but can be counteracted or modified and made more unctuous by adding a warm salad oil dressing.
- Beans – the irritant properties of most beans can be reduced by boiling them. Spices such as cumin, cayenne and asafoetida are helpful antidotes.
- Dairy – spices can be used to antidote and reduce its damp and mucus-forming Gunas. Milk can be heated and antidoted with ginger, cardamom and cinnamon.
- Spices are useful and should be chosen according to your Dosha type to make a meal more digestible, with more heating spices for Vata and Kapha and more cooling spices for Pitta.

• Toast and rice cakes – add butter and honey or a dip of hummus or guacamole to reduce their dryness and Vata aggravation, thus adding moisture and unctuousness.
• Curry is hot and pungent but reducing the heating spices and adding yoghurt, cooling herbs and spices such as coriander reduces the heat and makes it less Pitta-aggravating.

This is a useful way of being able to adapt foods for each of the Doshas. However, it is still better to follow the guidelines for your Dosha type. Using antidoting as a way to continue eating foods that you know don't really suit you is not recommended.

A meal with all tastes

Ayurveda recommends incorporating all six tastes into a meal. This needs to be done with care, balancing and blending flavours to create a tasty meal that suits our digestion.

We can design a meal that includes a selection of component parts to incorporate the six tastes. This enables a meal to easily include a variety of tastes that can cater for people with different Doshas and tastes. The classic Asian curry is a good example of this. Combining rice, mild vegetable 'curries', dhal, greens, pickles, cooling yoghurt and spices including salt, pepper and coriander enables people to select dishes, garnishes and quantities to match their individual needs.

Often a traditional British meal may be missing one or more tastes. For instance, a roast chicken dinner served with a selection of root and green leafy vegetables lacks the sour taste. In this example we can become creative by adding a simple appetiser of grated ginger, apple cider vinegar and salt or a small spoonful of sauerkraut at the beginning of the meal to aid digestion. Alternatively, we could cheat a little and add a dessert course of baked apples (sweet, astringent & sour) to incorporate the missing taste.

Interestingly, the traditional ploughman's lunch of bread, cheese, pickles, an apple and a pint of beer, with a 'twist' of salt, incorporates all six tastes.

We can also create a single dish incorporating all tastes. Single-dish meals work well, especially when you are eating on your own.

Kitchari is made from split mung beans (sweet and astringent), basmati rice (sweet), ghee (sweet) and the spices ginger (pungent and sweet), mustard (pungent), cumin (pungent), coriander (pungent and sweet), turmeric (bitter, pungent and astringent) and salt. We can then add some lime juice as a garnish to the finished dish for the sour taste. If we serve this with a small portion of a green vegetable such as kale (astringent, sweet and bitter) or Swiss chard (astringent and bitter), we add more astringent and bitter taste to the final dish.

Roasted vegetables could include carrots (sweet and pungent), squash (sweet), garlic (pungent, sweet, sour, bitter and astringent), tomatoes (sweet and sour) and some herbs and spices – basil (pungent), rosemary (pungent and bitter), black pepper (pungent) and salt. If served with some crumbled feta cheese (sweet and sour) and an astringent green vegetable, this gives us the six tastes.

Broccoli soup made from onion (pungent and sweet), celery (astringent, sweet and sour), broccoli (astringent and sweet) and garlic (pungent, sweet, sour, bitter and astringent), flavoured with cider vinegar (sour), salt and pepper (pungent), gives us all six tastes in one dish.

We can add garnishes and accompaniments to dishes and meals to provide additional taste and flavour to suit each Dosha. The options are endless and include:

- a swirl of yoghurt or sour cream – sweet and sour
- toasted nuts and seeds – sweet
- a little crumbled cheese – sweet and sour
- a scattering of fresh herbs: pungent coriander, parsley or sweet mint
- a splash of lemon juice – sour
- the addition of a few chilli flakes – pungent
- a small treat of bitter dark chocolate at the end of a meal
- a few roasted fennel seeds (sweet and pungent) at the end of a meal.

Adapting recipes:

Adapting a recipe using healthier ingredients

There are many ways of changing the way we eat, and one is to adapt recipes. This could be done by replacing all or some of the meat with plant-based alternatives; making burgers from lentils, nuts or mushrooms or replacing a shop-bought or take-away pizza with a homemade one. Some people are more confident than others at adapting recipes; for example, cottage pie could be adapted by replacing some or all of the meat with lentils or mushrooms. We can also add some finely chopped vegetables, carrots or tomatoes to bulk it out and replace the mashed potato top with mashed cauliflower or sweet potato. These subtle changes can also be used to adapt a recipe for each Dosha.

Adapting a recipe with healthier cooking methods

We can also adapt how we cook food by using healthier cooking methods. We can poach or oven-bake fish, steam vegetables, poach, scramble or boil an egg, use a pressure cooker to cook beans or use a rice cooker for rice or kitchari.

A rice cooker can be a useful kitchen appliance, especially for cooking kitchari. When you are tired or short of time you can use it to combine all the ingredients and provide an easy, healing meal without any effort.

Menu ideas

Small dishes – a handful of ideas

These dishes below are suitable for all Doshas as part of a balanced diet. You can modify the recipe for your dominant Dosha.

• Soup – vegetables; optionally add pulses, chicken broth, miso
• Vegetables – roasted root vegetables (limited for Kapha), stir fry, ratatouille (reduce tomatoes for Pitta), sautéed with ghee and spices
• Pâtés, dips & terrines – avocado, beetroot, mushroom, aubergine
• Serve with crudité vegetables. These can be useful for a packed lunch
• Salads – mixed salad using cooked grains, greens and protein ingredients together (known as a buddha bowl), tabbouleh (try with riced cauliflower or quinoa), with wilted greens, pressed salad, blanched salad. Best eaten in summertime for lunch
• Beans and pulses – falafel, hummus, dhal
• Eggs – poached, omelette, frittata, flan, cocotte. Best eaten at lunch
• Cheese – halloumi, fresh soft cheese, tofu with salad or vegetables. Best eaten at lunch.

Smaller meals are tasty and appetising and enable us to leave the table feeling lighter.

Large dishes – a handful of ideas

These dishes are suitable for all Doshas as part of a balanced diet. You can modify the recipe for your dominant Dosha.

Composite dishes – a meal in itself, using vegetables to replace meat. Examples might be curry (mild for Pitta), stews, stuffed vegetables, chilli non-carne with rice (mild for Pitta), bakes (with a crusty topping) or stir-fry vegetables with rice.

Grains – experiment with alternative flours to wheat to make pancakes, crêpes or flans with vegetable fillings, and pasta with vegetable-based sauces. Choose grains suitable for your Dosha type.

Rice – used as the grain option with vegetables or as a composite dish such as risotto.

Chicken – roast, poached, sautéed or chicken bone broth.

Breakfast

Vata

It is good to include a warm dish for a Vata breakfast to balance and pacify Vata at the start of the day. A light to moderate meal could include:

- Seasonal fruit or warm stewed fruit (sweet or sour)
- Cooked grain porridge with milk of your choice,

sweet spices, natural sweetener (and a little ghee optional)
• Herbal tea

Pitta
Pitta benefit from having a larger breakfast to avoid getting hungry until lunchtime.
• Seasonal sweet fruit or warm stewed fruit
• Cooked grain porridge in winter or a raw cereal (granola or muesli) in summer with milk and natural sweetener
• Wholemeal toast with butter and conserve
• Herbal tea

Kapha
Kapha benefit from having a light later breakfast or nothing at all, unless you are physically active or hungry.

• Seasonal fruit or warm stewed fruit and Ginger tea

Packed lunches

One option for lunch, especially if you are working, is to prepare and take your own picnic or packed lunch. Try to avoid a diet comprised solely of sandwiches made with wheat-based bread. Have fun being creative to include a variety of dishes – look at the suggestions above. You might like to invest in a Tiffin or Bento Box to contain your own creative dish or invest in a vacuum food flask to enjoy a warming soup, dhal or kitchari. This is often cheaper and healthier than relying on the choices available when you are out and about. It's even better if you can enjoy having your picnic in a peaceful setting to give you a real break.

Snacking

If you are going to have a snack, think about healthy snack ideas and ensure that there is something healthy at hand in the kitchen cupboard, office drawer or car to avoid reaching for the biscuit tin!

- Healthy snack ideas: a piece of fruit, a small handful of nuts or dates, bliss balls or crudité vegetables with a little dip.
- If you crave something sweet, try a cinnamon and liquorice tea, or opt for a home-made muffin or flapjack made with a natural sweetener.
- If it's a cold day and you need warming up, try a spicy milk drink with ginger, turmeric and cinnamon.
- Avoid processed snacks, biscuits and confectionery that are often high in calories and low in nutrients.
- Sometimes snacking can be an indication of thirst rather than hunger, so it is useful to ask yourself the question, 'Am I hungry or am I thirsty'?

14. Putting It All Together

How do we put it all together?

Doshas

Perhaps a good place to start is with your Dosha. If you have completed the Dosha questionnaires in Appendix 1 you will know what your Dosha Prakriti and Vikriti are. Or maybe it's left you feeling a bit confused. It is not always easy to evaluate ourselves. Sometimes it helps to ask an Ayurveda practitioner to assist you with this.

We generally eat seasonally and use the Dosha Prakriti diet for each season when we are healthy and well. When we are a mixed Dosha type, we adjust this accordingly, as detailed above. This is our diet for life.

When we are showing signs of imbalance (Vikriti), we use a short-term stricter diet to bring the Dosha that is most aggravated back into balance. This is usually your Dosha Prakriti, your strongest Dosha. However, in today's world it could also be Vata Dosha that is most aggravated. We live in a very Vata-aggravating world with high stress, insomnia and anxiety, too much time on the computer, on our phones and watching TV, which can all leave us feeling Vata-aggravated, even when Vata isn't our dominant Dosha.

Agni, our digestive fire

Could your digestion do with some improvements? Do you suffer from wind, bloating, acidity or constipation? If so, it's worth going back and reviewing the section on improving Agni and trying some of the recommendations. How you feel after a meal is a guide as to whether your diet suits you.

Ama

Are you showing symptoms of Ama? Again, if so, go back and look at the section on Ama, particularly the causes and signs of Ama and the Anti-Ama diet.

It is also important to remember that Ayurveda is as much about how you eat as what you eat. So, you might like to review the section on general advice as well.

Any change to the way you eat needs to take account of your budget, lifestyle and motivation for wanting to change. I would encourage you to buy good-quality ingredients, eat more plant-based foods, eat more seasonal, locally produced food, and cook more of your own meals if you're not already doing this.

Our style of cooking is influenced from our childhood and normally by how well our primary carer cooked. We are all influenced by our own age, generation and background. Change doesn't have to be radical; just take one step at a time, one meal at a time. It could be cooking a home-made pizza or some bliss balls with your children, or trying a new vegetarian recipe at the weekend when you hopefully have a bit more time to enjoy it. If you know that your diet could do with improving, then become inspired to make some positive changes. What is important is how you feel when you have finished eating; you should feel satisfied and energised, not dissatisfied by a meal that is too light or too heavy. It's about keeping everything in balance.

Recipes

Kitchari

If there's one meal that you are encouraged to make a staple, it's the Ayurveda classic kitchari, which is balancing and cleansing and easy to digest. It is Sattvic, helps to remove Ama and is suitable for all three Doshas. Make it a regular lunch or supper dish to aid your digestion, as well as using it as a wonderful convalescent meal. This is a simple version of this recipe that serves two people.

Ingredients:

50g split mung beans (mung dhal), yellow or green (well rinsed)
100g basmati rice or quinoa (well rinsed)
1 teaspoon ghee or oil
¼–½ teaspoon each of ground cumin, ginger and turmeric, plus a little rock salt and black pepper
800ml water

Method:

1. Heat the ghee over a medium heat in a saucepan.
2. Add the spices and cook for a minute, then add a little water to avoid burning them.

3. Add the rice, dhal and the rest of the water and bring to the boil. Cover and simmer (with gentle bubbles on the surface) for about 20 minutes until soft, adding more water if required.

The end result should be soft and moist, similar to a risotto.

Note: Alternatives and Adaptations

A more traditional cooking method is to use fresh herbs and whole spices, which are more Sattvic: 1” of fresh peeled and chopped ginger and turmeric and 1 teaspoon of cumin seeds.

Lightly cook the cumin seeds in the heated ghee until they start to brown, become fragrant and start to ‘pop’, which takes about 1 minute. Be careful not to burn the seeds, then add the ginger and turmeric before adding a little water.

If you have them in your kitchen cupboard, further spices can be added, including mustard seeds, coriander, cardamom and asafoetida.

A quick alternative method of cooking for when you are short of time and energy is to use ground spices and put all the ingredients together into a rice cooker, stir and let it cook itself. Stir well before serving.

Garnish with coriander, grated coconut or a squeeze of lemon.

Adapting the classic recipe, it can be turned into an even more delicious dish by the addition of some cooked vegetables – carrots, squash, broccoli, spinach or kale.

A rice mini cooker is ideal to use for making kitchari for one person, away from home, in the office, or when travelling, especially if you have a delicate digestion. I find a ratio of 40g split mung beans, 80g of rice and 400ml of water with the spices and ghee works well to make 1 large or 2 small portions.

Ghee

Ghee made from cow's milk is highly valued in Ayurveda, is considered to be the best fat for the body and is highly nutritious. In the UK we know it as clarified butter. Ghee is traditionally made by heating unsalted organic butter until it becomes a golden liquid.

Ayurveda considers it a *Rasayana*, a rejuvenating and longevity-promoting food. The gentle cooking of butter enables the milk solids to be removed, leaving the sweet-tasting oil.

In small doses it is easy to digest and is considered balancing for all three Doshas. Ghee pacifies Pitta and Vata and is acceptable in moderation for Kapha. It should be used with caution if you have Ama or high cholesterol or suffer from obesity.

At first, try making 1–2 blocks of butter. However, if you start using ghee in all your cooking, you may want to make up larger quantities.

Ingredients:

250g – 500g unsalted butter – only use organic

Utensils:

You will need a medium saucepan and a clean, dry jam jar or two. It is also good if you have some muslin cloth, but a piece of ordinary plain cotton will do. Ensure that all your cooking utensils and jars are clean and sterile before you begin in order to avoid the risks of contamination or of mould forming.

One method for sterilising the jars is given below.

Sterilising:

- Preheat oven to 160 °C.
- Wash jars and lids in hot soapy water and then rinse them well.
- Place the jars on a baking tray and put into the oven for 10 minutes.
- Soak the lids in boiling water for a few minutes.

Method:

1. Melt the butter in a pan on medium–low heat. Then reduce the heat to low. It will foam and bubble.
2. Remove the foam during cooking. At first, it is good to remove the foam as it cooks, so that you can see what is going on underneath. However, one can with practice judge when the ghee is nearly ready and remove the foam at that stage.
3. Solids will form, and eventually sink to the bottom and start to turn brown. The ghee will begin to become golden or light brown and sweet smelling.
4. Stir the ghee occasionally to prevent it from sticking (some methods say don't stir it but both ways work).
5. It is ready when all the solids have fallen to the

bottom and the ghee isn't spitting anymore and has a good golden colour that is clear, transparent and not cloudy.

6. Allow to cool slightly, then pour the liquid ghee into clean, dry, sterilised jars. If you have some muslin, you can filter the ghee at this stage, preventing any residual foam or floating solids from mixing in with the ghee (a tiny bit will be okay).
7. When you pour the ghee into the jars, do so within a large bowl or basin – this means that if the glass jar breaks it doesn't create a glorious mess! But if this does happen, discard and start again.
8. Leave the ghee to cool a little, which will take about 10–15 minutes, and then seal the jars with a lid and leave to set.

Note: There are plenty of videos you can watch online if you are a little unconfident the first time you make ghee. Be careful not to burn it.

How long will it take to cook?

If you are prepared to stand over the ghee and you are making a small amount (1–2 blocks of butter) then you can cook it at a medium to low heat in around 30–45 minutes.

However, for larger amounts, or if you have the time, cook it at a very low temperature, which will take about two hours.

Storage:

If cooked long enough, it can in theory be stored indefinitely in a cool, dry place away from direct sunlight. However, I recommend using it within three to six months. Ghee does not need refrigeration. Its medicinal properties are said to improve with age. Don't ladle out the ghee with a wet spoon or allow any water to get into the container, as this will create the conditions for bacteria to grow and spoil the ghee.

Bone broth

Bone broth is not a modern idea but is a classic Ayurveda recipe that has been known for thousands of years; it is healing, nourishing and easy to digest. It is now coming back into our consciousness and is especially good for curing a leaky gut. It is recommended for when we are not feeling well; think of it as a replacement for Grandma's homemade chicken soup! It gives us the nutritional benefits of the meat without the flesh that is heavy and hard to digest and that results in forming Ama. There are many variations, but here is a simple chicken broth recipe that doesn't take too long to cook.

Ingredients:
4 organic chicken wings or drumsticks + chicken feet if available
75g fresh root ginger – chopped
5 kaffir lime leaves
2 lemongrass stalks – bruised
1 teaspoon black peppercorns
1 teaspoon salt

Method:
1. Put all the ingredients into a large pot with 1½ litres of water.
2. Let it come to the boil and simmer with the lid on for 3–4 hours.
3. Stir occasionally.
4. After 1 hour, gently take the chicken meat off the bones to expose the bones for cooking.

5. When cooking is complete, strain the stock through a fine sieve to create a clear broth. The cooked broth can be cooled and stored in batches in the freezer to use as a nourishing and healing thin soup, as the foundation to a soup recipe or as stock in cooking.

The chicken meat can be used for another dish or added back into the broth to make chicken soup.

A pressure cooker reduces the cooking time.

Apple Bliss Balls

Bliss Balls are always a treat and there are many recipes available online and in recipe books. The fresh apple makes this recipe light and moist, though you could use dried apple if preferred. This recipe makes about 25 bliss balls.

Ingredients:

100g dates (no stones)
50g ground almonds
30g walnuts
1 dessert apple (peeled and cored)
1 teaspoon powdered cinnamon
20g cocoa nibs (optional)
For coating: chopped nuts, or desiccated coconut, or cocoa powder (whatever you have to hand)

Method:

1. Blitz all the ingredients in the food processor using the S-blade until the ingredients bind together – about 1–2 minutes. If you're adding the cocoa nibs, you can do so at the end so that they still keep their texture and are not completely melted into the mix.
2. Scoop a teaspoon of the mixture and roll it between the palms of your hands to create little balls.
3. Roll the balls in the coating – this stops them sticking together.
4. Store them in an airtight container or in the fridge or freezer.

Ayurveda glossary of Sanskrit terms

Sanskrit is an ancient and complex language in which words and phrases can often have more than one interpretation and indeed more than one spelling. This glossary explains some of the terms used in this book.

Agni – our digestive fire. It relates to both physical and mental digestion:

- ***Jathara Agni*** – the digestion of food in the stomach
- ***Pancha Bhuta Agni*** – enzyme function in the liver, with one Agni for each of the five elements (see *Pancha Maha Bhuta* later in this glossary)
- ***Dhatu Agni*** – digestion at a cellular level. There are seven groups of Agnis, one for each Dhatu (level of body tissue).

Ahara – diet or food.

Ama – a by-product of toxins in our digestive tract from food that has not been fully digested, absorbed or evacuated. Ama prevents the body from functioning well and is a major cause of disease. We can observe the presence of Ama on our tongue when it is not clear and clean.

Chikitsa – medicine, treatment or therapy.

Dhatus – parts of the structural anatomy of the body, which Ayurveda perceives in a different way to modern medicine. The body is made up of seven Dhatus or body tissues from the food we eat, with each Dhatu nourishing the next level of Dhatu.

Doshas – the three intelligent principles that govern the functioning of the body.
They are affected by our diet and lifestyle, our environment, seasons and time and, when aggravated, can cause disease in the physical body:

- ***Vata*** – manages movement in the body
- ***Pitta*** – manages transformation and digestion in the body
- ***Kapha*** – provides structure and lubrication to the body.

We have all three Doshas within us. However, we usually have a predominant Dosha that will determine our physical and mental disposition.

Gunas – ten pairs of qualities that can be used to describe everything in nature:

Gunas	**Opposite Gunas**
Cold	Hot
Wet/oily	Dry
Heavy	Light
Gross	Subtle
Dense	Flowing
Static	Mobile

Dull	Sharp
Soft	Hard
Smooth	Rough
Cloudy	Clear

Kitchari – a classic Ayurveda recipe made from rice and split mung beans (mung dal) with digestive spices.

Pancha Karma – a specialist therapy treatment of strong internal and external purification therapies carried out in a clinical environment to cleanse the body and balance the Doshas. These therapies can be helpful to promote health and longevity and to help recovery from specific diseases.

Pancha Maha Bhuta – the five great elements ('Pancha' means 'five'):

Ether/Space	Akasha
Air	Vayu
Fire	Agni
Water	Jala
Earth	Prthivi

Ayurveda is based on the philosophy that cosmic energy manifests as the Pancha Maha Bhuta. Everything in the universe, including our bodies, can be classified using these five energies through the Doshas and the food we eat.

Prakriti – is our unique Dosha constitutional type or natal constitution – our unique genetic blueprint. Prakriti identifies how we function when we are healthy and balanced. We can identify our Dosha nature by observing our physical and mental characteristics.

Prana – pure energy, the intelligent principle of energy in the universe, our vital life force. Prana comes from our breath, fresh foods and pure water.

Rajas – the cosmic quality of energy, action, movement and dispersion; it supports activity in life. We seek to reduce our use of Rajasic foods that over-stimulate the body and mind – for example, coffee and white sugar.

Rasa – the Sanskrit word for 'taste'. Ayurveda identifies six tastes: sweet, sour, salt, pungent, bitter and astringent.

Sātmya – the principle of habituation and our ability to adapt to our environment. We are predisposed to our place of origin; its local foods, climate, habits and culture. We can struggle to adapt to changes brought about by moving to new foreign environments, or by adapting to imported or modern foods that are not part of our heritage.

Sattva – the cosmic quality of purity, light and clarity; it is the true state of the mind. Foods that support Sattva are pure, fresh and as natural as possible.

Srotamsi (plural) or ***Srotas*** (singular) – the 16 channels of the body used for internal communication and digestion. These channels include those connected to the breath, food and liquid; channels linked to each of the Dhatus; the mind; and for women two additional channels relating to menstruation and lactation.

Tamas – the cosmic quality of inertia, darkness and dullness. We should seek to avoid Tamasic foods, including processed ready meals, fried foods and reheated food that have no Prana or vitality.

Vikriti – identifies when we are out of balance or dis-eased – when our natural Prakriti Dosha balance is distorted or obscured by Dosha imbalances.

Appendix 1
Dosha Questionnaire

Prakriti questionnaire

To determine your Prakriti, or life-long constitution, base your answers on what has been consistent over your life, especially looking back to when you were younger, in childhood and before any long-term health issues, to establish your constitution from birth.

Tick the box that seems most appropriate to you and add up the numbers for Vata, Pitta and Kapha to see which is your dominant Dosha (or Doshas).

It is often difficult to determine your Prakriti or Vikriti just from a questionnaire, and consulting with an Ayurvedic practitioner can often give you a better idea and avoid personal bias.

Observation	*Vata*	*V*	*Pitta*	*P*	*Kapha*	*K*
Body frame	Slim		Medium		Large	
Body weight	Light		Medium		Heavy	
Skin	Thin, cold, dry, rough		Warm, oily, smooth, freckled		Pale, cool, soft, oily	
Hair	Thin, brittle, dry, coarse		Fine, red, grey or bald		Thick, oily, glossy	

Observation	*Vata*	*V*	*Pitta*	*P*	*Kapha*	*K*
Face	Small, oval, thin, irregular features		Medium, prominent features		Round, large	
Tongue	Narrower than teeth, thin tip		Same width as teeth, oval-shaped tip		Wider than teeth, thick, round tip	
Hands	Small, long fingers		Medium, symmetrical		Large, thick short fingers	
Fingernails	Dry, rough, brittle, break easily		Pink, flexible		White, strong, smooth, thick	
Digestion	Variable, internal gas, allergies		Strong, quick, able to digest almost anything, acidity, burning		Slow but steady, heaviness	
Eating habits	Irregular, grazes or misses meals		Never misses a meal, gets hungry		Love food, overeats, can miss breakfast	
Food sensitivities	Astringent drying legumes, cabbage		Onions, oily foods, Solanaceae (tomatoes, potatoes, peppers, chillies)		Dairy, sugar, white flour	
Thirst	Changeable, drinks a lot		Gets thirsty		Doesn't get thirsty	
Faeces	Sparse, hard, dry, constipation		Soft, oily, loose, diarrhoea		Large heavy stools, sluggish, sticky	
Sweat	Little with no smell		Gets sweaty, strong smell		Moderate, neutral smell	

Observation	*Vata*	*V*	*Pitta*	*P*	*Kapha*	*K*
Energy level	Active, erratic, stops and starts, tires easily		Average, determined		Slow but steady, good stamina, slow in starting	
Sensitivity to environment	Likes warmth, dislikes wind and cold		Likes coolness, dislikes heat		Likes sun and wind, dislikes cold and damp	
Resistance to disease	Weak immune system, variable		Average, gets infections		Strong immune system, slow to get ill, slow to get well	
Speech	Fast, talkative, unclear, rambling		Sharp, clear, penetrating, convincing		Slow, taciturn, succinct	
Mental nature	Hyperactive, changeable, indecisive		Competitive, intense, critical, analytical		Steady, placid, methodical	
Emotional attitude	Lively, anxious, fearful, talks about feelings		Perceptive, intolerant, angry, dominating, impatient		Resilient, stable, greedy, sentimental, attached	
Sleep	Light, irregular, restless		Moderate, broken but will get back to sleep		Long and deep sleep, hard to wake up	
Menstruatio n (for women)	Cycle 26–28 days, light flow 2–3 days duration, irregular, PMS		Cycle 28 days, heavy flow, 3–5 days duration, bright red blood		Cycle 28–30 days, 4–7 days duration, medium flow thicker and paler	
TOTALS	**VATA**		**PITTA**		**KAPHA**	

Vikriti questionnaire

To determine your Vikriti or current constitution, showing where your Doshas may be out of balance from your Prakriti, base your answers on how you are now, including any changes brought about by your current lifestyle and health.

Tick the box that seems most appropriate to you and add up the numbers for Vata, Pitta and Kapha to see which is your current dominant Dosha (or Doshas).

Observation	*Vata*	*V*	*Pitta*	*P*	*Kapha*	*K*
Body frame	Slim		Medium		Large	
Body weight	Light, difficult to put on weight		Medium		Heavy, prone to weight gain	
Skin	Thin, cold, dry, rough, prominent veins		Warm, oily, smooth, acne, inflamed		Pale, cool, soft, oily	
Hair	Thin, brittle, dry, coarse		Fine, red, grey or bald easily		Thick, oily, glossy	
Face	Small, oval, thin, irregular features		Medium, prominent features		Round, large	
Tongue	Narrower than teeth, thin tip		Same width as teeth, oval-shaped tip		Wider than teeth, thick, round tip	
Hands	Small, long fingers		Medium, symmetrical		Large, thick, short fingers	

Observation	*Vata*	*V*	*Pitta*	*P*	*Kapha*	*K*
Fingernails	Dry, rough, brittle, break easily, bitten		Pink, flexible		White, strong, thick	
Digestion	Variable, internal gas – wind and bloating, allergies, anorexia		Strong, quick, able to digest almost anything, acidity, burning		Slow but steady, heaviness, bloating	
Eating habits	Irregular, grazes or misses meals		Never misses a meal, gets hungry		Loves food, overeats, can miss breakfast, emotional eating	
Food sensitivities	Astringent drying foods – legumes, cabbage		Onions, oily foods, Solanaceae vegetables		Dairy, sugar, white flour	
Thirst	Changeable, drinks a lot		Gets thirsty		Doesn't get thirsty	
Faeces	Sparse, dry, hard, constipation		Soft, oily, loose, diarrhoea		Large heavy stools, sluggish, can have mucus in stool	
Sweat	Little with no smell		Gets sweaty, hot strong smell		Moderate, neutral smell	
Energy level	Active, erratic, stops and starts, tires easily, exhaustion		Average, determined, exhaustion from over-thinking		Slow but steady, good stamina, exhaustion from excess weight	

Observation	*Vata*	*V*	*Pitta*	*P*	*Kapha*	*K*
Sensitivity to environment	Likes warmth, dislikes cold and wind		Likes coolness, dislikes heat		Likes sun and wind, dislikes cold and damp	
Resistance to disease	Variable, weak immune system		Average, gets infections		Strong immune system, slow to get ill, slow to get well	
Disease tendencies	Pain, mental disorders, eating disorders, insomnia, dry wheezing, diseases of nervous system		Fever, infections, inflammatory heart diseases, rashes		Respiratory diseases, mucus, oedema, obesity, stagnation	
Mental nature	Hyperactive, changeable, indecisive, impulsive		Competitive, intense, critical, analytical		Slow, placid, methodical	
Emotional attitude	Lively, anxious, fearful, worries, depression		Perceptive, intolerant, angry, dominating, frustrated, temper tantrums		Resilient, stable, depression, grief, calm, greedy, unresponsiv eness	
Sleep	Light, irregular, insomnia, restless		Moderate, broken		Long and deep, hard to wake up, drowsiness	
Menstruatio n (for women)	Cycle 26–28 days, light flow 2–3 days duration, irregular, PMS		Cycle 28 days, heavy flow, 3–5 days duration, bright red blood		Cycle 28–30 days, 4–7 days duration, medium flow thicker and paler	
TOTALS	**VATA**		**PITTA**		**KAPHA**	

Appendix 2
Seasonal British fruit & vegetables

	SPRING March - May	SUMMER June - August	AUTUMN September - November	WINTER December - February
Fruit	Rhubarb	Apricot Blueberries Cherries Currants Gooseberries Peaches Plums Raspberries Strawberries	Apples Blackberries Damsons Elderberries Figs Pears Plums Quince Sloes	Apples Pears
Veget-ables	Asparagus Jersey Royal Potatoes Purple sprouting broccoli Radishes Savoy cabbage Spinach Spring greens Spring onions Watercress	Aubergine Beetroot Broad beans Broccoli Capsicum peppers Carrots Courgettes Cucumber Fennel Fresh peas Garlic Globe artichokes Green beans Lettuce New potatoes Radishes	Beetroot Capsicum peppers Carrots Celeriac Celery Fennel Field mushrooms Globe artichokes Kale Leeks Lettuce Marrows Onions Potatoes Pumpkin Rocket	Beetroot Brussels sprouts Cabbage Cauliflower Celeriac Celery Chicory Jerusalem artichokes Kale Leeks Parsnips Potatoes Red cabbage Swedes Turnips

	SPRING March - May	SUMMER June - August	AUTUMN September - November	WINTER December - February
		Rocket Runner beans Salad leaves Salad onions Tomatoes Watercress	Squashes Sweetcorn Tomatoes Watercress	

Bibliography

Ayurveda Medicine for Westerners volume 1
Anatomy and Physiology in Ayurveda by Vaidya Atreya Smith 2013
Published by EIVS GmbH

Ayurveda Medicine for Westerners volume 2
Pathology, Diagnosis and Treatment Approaches in Ayurveda by Vaidya Atreya Smith 2014
Published by EIVS GmbH

Ayurveda Medicine for Westerners volume 3
Clinical Protocols and Treatment in Ayurveda by Vaidya Atreya Smith 2015
Published by EIVS GmbH

Textbook of Ayurveda Volume 1
Fundamental Principles by Vasant Lad 2002
The Ayurvedic Press New Mexico

Ayurveda and Panchakarma
The science of healing and rejuvenation By Sunil V Joshi MD (Ayu) 1997
Published by Lotus Press, USA

Food for Life
by Tim Spector 2022
Published by Penguin UK

Mediterranean
Naturally nutritious recipes from the world's healthiest diet by Susie Theodorou 2018
Published by Kyle Books UK

Sanskrit English Dictionary
By Sir M. Monier-Williams 2006
published by Oxford University Press UK

Bibliography of classical texts:

Caraka Samhita volumes 1–7
by Dr R Sharma and Vadya Bhagwan Dash 2015
Published by Chowkhamba Sanskrit Series Office, Varanasi India

Astanga Hrdayam volumes 1–3
Translated by Prof. K.R. Srikantha Murthy 10th edition 2014
Published by Chowkhamba Krishnadas Academy, Varanasi India

Digestive teas:

Sebastian Pole is the founder of Pukka Tea and is a clinical practitioner using a blend of Ayurveda, Chinese and Western herbal medicine. The expert on digestive tea.

Cleanse Nurture Restore with Herbal Tea
by Sebastian Pole 2016
Published by Francis Lincoln, UK

Other links:

1. Ayurveda Professional Association
https://apa.uk.com
The APA is the largest Ayurveda organisation for Ayurveda in the UK. They can help you find the Ayurveda Professional best suited to your unique needs.

2. Coeliac UK
https://www.coeliac.org.uk
Coeliac UK is the charity for people who need to live without gluten. It provides independent, trustworthy advice and support so that people can live well, gluten free.

3. Environmental Working Group
https://www.ewg.org
The Environmental Working Group produces an annual *Shopper's Guide to Pesticides in Produce* and the *Clean Fifteen* and *Dirty Dozen* lists.

4. Bristol Stool Chart
There isn't one definitive website for this, but if you search Bristol Stool Chart on the internet you will find a downloadable chart.

Printed in Great Britain
by Amazon

60898651R00127